MW00440451

BRAINSURGEON
wings on an angel - clouds on a ghost

DR. MARK WEISSMAN

Copyright © 2015 Dr. Mark Weissman.

All Rights Reserved. No part(s) of this book may be reproduced, distributed or transmitted in any form, or by any means, or stored in a database or retrieval systems without prior expressed written permission of the author of this book.

ISBN: 978-1-62217-418-8

Table of Contents

PROLOGUE AND A GOOD WAY TO START, MAYBE

I'VE SPENT A LOT OF time thinking about thinking.

When I started medical school, I took the usual premedical courses, including calculus and the submarine sandwiches of chemistry, physics, and biology. They never really impressed me as ways to make listening to a stethoscope with greater clearing and meaning. The books were always very dramatic to look at, but I had trouble understanding what looked like ancient Egyptian papyrus inside.

When I was fifteen years old and a sophomore in high school, I was visiting with a friend of mine living in our neighborhood. It happens that his older brother was a first-year medical school student and was spending the weekend in Brooklyn. Remembering that I grew up in the middle earth of Brooklyn, like any average Hobbit, I decided that it wasn't a serious felony to search around the empty bedroom. My impression was that if I got physically closer to the medical books, I would clearly become smarter. On his desk was an open histology textbook. Histology is a study of the organs and cells of the body, and the explanations, to me, a high school sophomore, were totally lost.

I recall feeling faint and wondering how I could look at words in English and not understand a single sentence. My friend then entered his brother's room, where I was trying, unsuccessfully, to hide from my serious errors of judgment. My friend made it clear that not only should I not read any words from this sacrilegious text, but I should no longer enter his brother's room before I find myself encountered by locusts from the heaven's above. Eventually, I slowly learned that working is, at times, better than running.

At sixty-four years old, I found myself navigating an interesting conundrum. I planned to write an autobiography, but I wasn't certain how to deal with facts that were mostly forgotten or those facts I wish to forget.

Interestingly, friends, colleagues, and loved ones would often ask me when I was planning to retire. The answer was always a simple one because I thought I would either collapse and die while working in the operating room (OR) or I'd wind up with some illness that impaired me and kept me from working as a neurosurgeon. Retirement was never an issue dealing with my age or wealth. If my health was good and my family was thriving, I would continue to work until my wife threw me out of the house.

It so happened that three months after my sixty-third birthday, I received a belated gift in the form of a cerebrovascular stroke.

This is my story. As in most stories, there is love and loss. I found a "calling" true to only me, and at its very best, it shared "wings on angels." I also found what I call my "ghost." This wasn't sweet, fluffy, and lighter than air. This was a cloud fueling a dark despair.

We may move around here and there, but for the most part, we'll start at the beginning.

GENEALOGY, WHO WE ARE AND WHY?

I HAD NO IDEA HOW difficult it was to define the genealogy of a family. As deep as you go, to try and dig up the roots it is quasi-impossible. Finding secure documents and clear and visible photographs goes well beyond the magic of the best Vegas magicians. Discussions among the aunts, uncles, moms and dads, brothers and sisters, and every other available living bloodline will not lead to a pleasant, orderly, and sentimental discussion at the dinner table.

My grandfather Jacob was born in Austria and subsequently moved to New York City (NYC). I know of siblings he had in Great Britain and Israel. Jacob's wife, my grandmother Dora, was probably born in Russia, but the mystery continues. My maternal grandfather, Arthur, and his wife Ida were born in Russia and then moved to NYC.

Jacob owned a small business and was a successful carpenter. He built cabinet freezers for butcher stores and cabinets for grocery marts. Arthur, my other grandfather, was a master tailor and worked in the garment district in NYC. He also owned a clothing store and designed fabric suits for men's ware.

Jacob passed away at the age of sixty-two from a massive heart attack. I was six years old at the time. Arthur was unhealthy and struggled with insulin-dependent diabetes for many years, forcing an early retirement.

During his later years, my father became a successful display manufacturer. He earned some Caesar Awards and other certificates for his display work. As is so often the case, his success came after many years of personal difficulty. Despite having had a coronary bypass, he continued to smoke and struggled with other ongoing problems. He grew up in a "tough" area of Brooklyn. His friends were troubled, and my father had a lot of difficulties getting his own life in order. My dad continued to carry a constant weight in his heart after he lost Jacob at a relatively young age. My dad struggled as an alcoholic, mixed with other abuses, until the final ten years of his life. He did beat this difficult challenge, but the payment was too high, and we lost him at the age of sixty-seven. Our nuclear family had its share of calamities.

My grandmother Ida was of strong Russian stock, and it was easy to call her a difficult woman. She was rare to smile and was physically abusive to my mom and her two siblings until their early teenage years.

My mother's marriage was mostly unhappy, even though they spent almost fifty years together. It took many years for my father to get healthy, and everyone in the vicinity had a price to pay. My mom was depressed and suffered from severe anxiety. She suffered from a variety of malignant anger and physical abuse. She would often scream in her home, such that close neighbors would hear her explosions, and if the police knew of her degree of physical abuse, she would have been arrested in this day and age. She punched us with fists to the head and face, and she beat us with wooden hangers. She tore hair out of our scalps, and she whipped us with my father's belts.

I have two siblings, one older and one younger sister. My older sister and I were most affected, physically and emotionally, and my younger sister suffered emotionally. Despite our many wounds, we all managed to succeed in our careers, but the consequences went deep and were quite functional.

Yes, this was all quite unhappy for my siblings and me, but there are greater and deeper meanings. In the 1950s and most of the 1960s, the mental health specialty was still developing. Psychoanalysis was slowly becoming more sophisticated, but pharmacology was still early in its development. Today, we have psychiatrists, clinical psychologists, an encyclopedia of neuroses and phobias you can find on your smartphone, and drugs that can treat every type of depression, insomnia, obsessive-compulsive disorder, and a cornucopia of diagnoses I have difficulty completing on my own.

My mom had some serious mental health issues, but she could never get past the horrible anger and depression that would last the entirety of her adult life. She had a schizoaffective disorder, that would be confused by most psychiatrists. When things were good or even great, she would find ongoing reasons for disillusionment. Here, I am describing the worst of the worse, but it was not a constant vacuum. She did have love to offer and was supportive in sharing much of her wisdom. She was ill, without many available remedies. Our parents had many crises, but they got healthier and turned out as far better grandparents than parents.

GOOD ENOUGH TO BE A DOCTOR?

ONE EVENING, I BECAME ILL with a fever, a rheumy nose, and a sore throat. I was seven years old. As it was after hours, physicians would visit their patients at their homes, and this was known as a house call. This continued through the 1960s and partly the 1970s. I had visited my pediatrician for routine examinations and vaccinations, always associated with a syringe and needle. I'm sure that my pediatrician didn't particularly look forward to any injections or other invasive forms of entertainment, but I, most certainly, needed to be an obvious hero. When the pediatrician examined me, I was particularly attentive to the way he looked at my eyes, nose, and ears. I eventually learned that there were odd tools to help in this examination. He would palpate, looking for secret things underneath the skin, and he seemed to be able to look at everything and see anything he needed to know. Occasionally, I would have the extreme good fortune of touching the jewel of all the jewels, my Aladdin's lamp. For me, this meant I got to use a stethoscope. It was scary to touch, and it felt almost religious, being around one. If you visited a hospital or a physician's office, you would almost, with certainty, find a stethoscope inside a side pocket or around the physician's neck. It was as equivalent as an actual MD (medical doctor).

My pediatrician was keen and quite stern. A smile never accompanied any hello or good-bye. He seemed to dress as if he were wearing a uniform. In winter, he would wear a heavy winter coat, cold or not, but in spring, he wore a raincoat, wet or dry. He wore a sports jacket with unicolor trousers, or a suit jacket with matching trousers. Over many years, I never saw him change the style of his shoes, which were black wingtips. He always wore black socks, a tie clasp, and a solid color shirt, usually white. As I got older and became more interested, wanting to know about being a doctor, talking with my pediatrician was like talking to the grim reaper.

My mom had a great idea and decided to purchase a junior doctor's gift. This was a toy gift, but some of the toys were fancier than others were. There was a black satchel with a red cross emblazoned on the front near the clasp. Within, I found a plastic and rubber stethoscope, a thermometer, a syringe, a plastic ophthalmoscope, a reflex knee-jerk hammer and an ear, nose, and throat mirror. I read every pamphlet I could find in order to learn something new, and the only gift I wanted was a doctor's kit, whether it was for a birthday, Hanukkah, Christmas (if I can confuse someone that I wasn't really Jewish), good exams at school, or any other reason worthy of my toy doctor's kit.

The doctor's kits became more sophisticated, and walking around my home with my satchel and a stethoscope around my neck, it became quite transcendental. I suppose that for a young lady of my age, with similar hobbies and fantasies, she would probably have had every conceivable Barbie doll available with all the appropriate accessories. I managed to never discuss my doctor apparel with my friends. Years later, I generously discussed my secrets when I, of course, had a real satchel hanging on my hand and wrist!

When I was a student in medical school, I recalled the first time I purchased my real satchel and all the instruments. I would then open one of my books that helped to explain how each different instrument worked, and over time, I would try all of them on my dad. This was one of my great memories.

Reading was my other great choice, and I read every novel I could find that had anything to do with medicine. I read about the Mayo brothers, Louis Pasteur, Marie and Pierre Curie, Banting and Best, those who identified insulin. There were many other books read, and I read mostly during my summer days off before I was too old and had to go to work.

Going through high school and college, I learned that becoming a doctor meant staying at the top of your class and pretty much with straight As. You earn a bachelor's degree when graduating college, and this generally means studying science or math. Some students may do very well in a foreign language or other social sciences, such as psychology or sociology. There exists a standardized exam called the Medical College Admissions Test. It is important to do well on this examination. Some students have published poetry or short stories, and this always helps to polish your existing curriculum vitae. Basically, you need very good grades, but if you are not straight A, that doesn't mean you will not be successful in finding your way to medical school.

Some European medical schools, all considered very accomplished, were tuition-free as long as the students earned admission and could speak the appropriate foreign language. Now, European universities are not free, but they are not nearly as expensive as American schools. Today, medical students can graduate college and medical school with $300,000 in debt, if not considerably more.

My feeling is that if this is the career you want and need, then you should do everything possible to make it happen. I am presenting the golden-ticket preparation. Not every student is good at everything and gets As consistently. Some are very good in the classwork but are more average in the standardized exams like the SATs, ACTs, MCATs, or the other exams that keep us awake at night. There are students that do very well on the standardized exams but not very well in the classrooms.

I recall a teacher I had in the sixth grade who told me that my penmanship was so bad that I would never succeed in school. Granted, my penmanship was never very readable, and after I became a physician, I purchased an ink seal with my name engraved to help the nurses with my horrible signature. After the sixth grade, I was placed into the special-progress class, which meant I skipped the eighth grade and went from seventh to ninth. I'm sure that my teacher was convinced it was a mistake and, despite my grades, I was still going to decline in years to come.

I've learned that your intellectual capacity changes over time and is determined by many issues. I've met extremely average students in high school and college who worked hard, found ways to get to medical school, and turned out to be brilliant students and physicians. It is not always obvious. I've met brilliant students going off to Ivy League medical schools who became average students and physicians.

If you believe in yourself, you will find a way. I've given lectures to premedical students who have told me that their grades weren't high enough for medical school, and they were thinking of doing something else in health care. Don't sell yourself short; believe in yourself and find your own map. You don't have to be the smartest or have any scholarships. There are other ways to open the doors.

EAGLE SCOUT, HIGH SCHOOL, LIFE, AND DEATH

BEFORE I STARTED COLLEGE, I became aware of a special program created through the Eagle Scout system administered by the Boy Scouts of America. This was a new way to prepare young men and women interested in finding a career in medicine. Several hospitals in NYC allowed these students to "shadow" physician residents and interns through a full workday. The students attended lectures prepared by the physicians and worked near the nursing staff. We worked closely with the physicians, seeing the patients on the ward and occasionally in the operating room (OR) and emergency room (ER).

I was fortunate enough to find a position at a large hospital in Brooklyn, but as inspired and excited as I was, it was magnified many times over by just walking through the corridors of a large city hospital. I spent many months during the summer working in the ER. At that time, family medicine and general medicine were the same and not yet considered a board-certified specialty. In the ER, we often found residents in family medicine or young general practitioners polishing their new skills. We also found semiretired physicians working in the ER to keep busy. These were retired surgeons, cardiologists, or internists. Most physicians working in an ER today are board-certified emergency room specialists. Because of my early entry into the hospital, I saw far more going on than many young medical students sitting in the lecture room.

One day, a six-year-old boy was brought to the ER by ambulance. He had been playing inside a large box near his garage door. For whatever reason, the child's father had not paid attention to the box, and he'd struck the box with his vehicle. I stood near a flurry of medical teams engaging in nonstop work before they were able to transfer the child to the OR. The next day, I learned that the child had died after his spleen had ruptured, causing massive bleeding. A six-year-old boy died because he was playing in a box near his garage door. He died because his father struck the box with a vehicle for no good reason. He died because the entirety of specialists and healthcare assistants were unable to save him, as often happens on television or in the movies. The doubt, uncertainty, and lack of logic in this event created what was probably my first real sense of unease in my own skin. I, of course, was as naïve as one can be at the age of sixteen, to begin to understand this lack of maturity, but it was all I had at the moment. This occurred almost fifty years ago, yet it is as clear as yesterday.

CHERISH IS THE WORD

ANOTHER DAY, WE WERE WAITING by the treatment rooms near the stretcher corridor when we all became nauseated by a fetid and foul scent. A middle-aged man was limping while oozing viscous sediment filled with flies and maggots. The leg was dying from gangrene, and at my age of sixteen, I was assured that I was encountering one of those unforgettable forget-me-nots. I will agree that I didn't faint or vomit, and clearly, this was the worst scent I'd ever encountered. That being said, I came to understand that there are dimensions of olfaction that are still hiding around the cosmos and continue to remain unknown to us.

The remedy for this particular illness involved placing a complete and thorough sterile scrub suit on (making me feel like a surgeon) followed by intensive cleansing of the gangrenous leg. The flies and maggots were killed using a tub of ether. I, of course, was thrilled with the idea of participating, and so a young RN and I prepared for our major procedure. Keeping awake with all the ether was the first real challenge. We then killed the maggots and cleaned the dead tissue out. We then placed a dermatologic ointment and covered everything with sterile bandages. The process took over two hours. When we completed our work, the patient was comfortable, wearing new pajamas, eating a cheese sandwich, and drinking a cup of coffee. He was very grateful for all our help, and this meant a lot to me. He was homeless, alcoholic, and suffered from psychiatric illness as well as other illnesses, such as diabetes. Just another day in paradise!

It continues to amaze me how many people are hungry, continue to struggle without adequate clothing or housing, and suffer from ongoing psychiatric disease.

Life, in all its wonder and miracle, can never overcome the chronic deletion of harm that has always been inherent to any viable system. I suspect that our philosophers need to guide us all to a grander utopia.

A PREMATURE EXAGGERATION

A YOUNG MAN IN HIS twenties presented to the ER with a relatively simple laceration in the forearm, one lovely summer day in Brooklyn. The physician in charge of the treatment room at the ER was a retired internist who was interested in working for a few extra hours to keep busy and earn some surplus income. He was a very pleasant and kind individual who spent a lot of additional time talking about medicine to a sixteen-year-old. He had an unusual hobby of keeping a stogie in his mouth, almost at all times. It was unlit when he was working in the treatment areas, but the stogie was there anyway. I liked spending time with him, and I learned quite a bit from talking with him. The physician in charge of the ER approached me and asked me if I wanted to place a few sutures in the laceration. He knew that I had assisted him and others with suturing, so he gave me the opportunity. For me, this was asking if I wanted to command a space mission to Mars.

I then prepared the treatment room and opened all the needed instruments. I completed a surgeon's cleansing of my hands and forearms and had an RN assist me in placing all the paraphernalia, such as a surgical hood, shoes, pants, and shirt. She helped me place my gloves on as well as the surgical mask. Surgical gloves carried a special texture, and I'm certain that if we can find a suitable scent we could sell it as cologne in Nordstrom. We can call it "Scent of a Surgeon's Hand" or "Heavenly Touch!" In all seriousness, I was prepped and ready to go. I cleansed the laceration after offering a little Novocain, and then we placed all the sterile drapes and final cleansing solution. After carefully administering more Novocain to make sure the patient was very comfortable, I chose the proper suture and began placing four independent, sequential stitches. The ER physician said everything looked great. We cleaned the treated area once again and then covered the area with a sterile dressing and adhesive tape. The RN gave instructions to the patient, and then the patient thanked me and called me doctor. He had no idea that I was hardly shaving!

My experience as a medical Eagle Scout was one of the most exciting times of my young career. It did create some difficulties. I found that I had no patience because I wanted to forget about college and start medical school now. In Europe, this is exactly how it works, but I didn't know the paradigm. In Europe, you go to what we would call high school in the United States. The European high school is more advanced than American high school. You earn a diploma called a baccalaureate at eighteen or nineteen years old. When you complete your baccalaureate, you decide your career plan, which could be medicine, math, biology, law, political science, foreign language, psychology, etc. You will learn a minimum of a master's degree or possibly a PhD or MD. There are no liberal colleges in Europe. For me, I consider this a negative, as most young people have no idea what careers to choose at eighteen or nineteen years old. This would have worked for me because I was prepared for this, and I graduated high school one month after turning seventeen. It wasn't because I was smarter; I was just ready to do it. My experience in the Eagle Scouts advanced me dramatically, and I had medicine on my mind for a very long time. Had I known of this system, I would have tried to start medical school in Europe. The humorous part is that I did study in Europe but for different reasons.

BROOKLYN COLLEGE, PREMEDICAL, FREE TUITION, EUROPE

I went to Brooklyn College, which is part of the City University of New York. At the time that I was matriculated, it was a free school with no tuition. This attracted a lot of students to this school. Other colleges that were part of the City University of New York were also tuition-free. New York City, free tuition, Jewish, Caucasian? Sounds great for me! The other side of that equation is called a premedical major. It seemed as if everyone wanted to go to medical school. Medical school cost about $20,000/year. There were some variabilities depending upon the type of school, but, for the most part, it was far less expensive than what we encounter these days.

After spending four years in college, with a major degree in biology and a completion of my premedical studies, I also completed my full share of liberal studies. Earning honors in all these divisions, I enjoyed only four subjects out of four years of college. Biochemistry and physiology were wonderful. I also took many courses in biology, chemistry, physics, and mathematics. Most of them were not fun, and neither were the extra pounds I added to my sorrowful butt while eating all that additional pizza.

My first psychology course was dismal. I didn't expect to take any other psychology courses in the near future or ever. When I was in my third year of college, a friend advised me to take a course in abnormal psychology. Even though I was dubious, I tried the course and found it to be one of the best courses of my college career. My next psychology course was called child psychology, and once again, I fell in love. With very high grades in these courses, I decided to go on to medical school and train to become a psychiatrist. It didn't quite work out that way, despite the pipe smoking, corduroy pants, and turtleneck sweaters. Most people who know me would imagine me developing a true allergy functioning as a psychiatrist.

Hard work and good grades throughout college did not accumulate a plethora of scholarships, and a mountain of debt did not seem particularly appealing. Throughout high school and college, French remained my second foreign language, and it served me well. At college, the students majoring in a foreign language were essentially female, and I was the only male, premedical science major. Studying all these romantic poems and novels in a French class cushioned with nothing but females learning French got my attention away from all the science.

Gathering information about studying in Europe, I found that it was tuition-free if you were admitted. There were plenty of Americans studying in Europe, and some loved living in a foreign country. The university was difficult, and it was not easy to do well without a serious amount of hard work. The medical school was longer than American medical schools, but you also earned an additional master's degree before completing your

MD diploma. There were Americans who did not like living in Europe and found every opportunity to get back to the United States.

Many Americans were attracted to studying at several of the universities in Belgium. Almost every examination was an oral exam, and most final exams were given at the end of the year, covering the entire year's work. The study was in the pyramid style, such that there were seven hundred students in the first year, but only two hundred students graduating at the end, earning the MD. Academics were like the Flying Wallendas balancing on a high wire over the Grand Canyon.

You needed to earn a master's degree in medical science as I previously mentioned, and the courses were very complicated and difficult to earn high grades. The paradigm for exam-taking was no different, whether the diploma was a master's or a doctorate. As an example, if you had five finals to pass at the end of the school year and you were successful passing four but failed one course, you would be required to take all five examinations again before the next academic year started. American medical schools are certainly not easy in the slightest sense of the word, but studying in Europe added a few additional cramps and strains. If an American student failed a course in medical school, the student would be assigned a tutor for supplemental preparation until the result was satisfactory.

The translation of the diploma in English was "doctor in medicine, surgery, obstetrics, and gynecology." It allowed for a large certificate occupying my office. Eventually, all my diplomas came down, replaced with more interesting artwork.

I've studied at American universities, including Ivy League, and I promise that getting through a European study in a foreign language cannot occur without effort. We learned how to study, even if it meant sucking fuel tanks of caffeine, nicotine, and the French equivalent of Benzedrine.

MORE FRENCH, AMPHITHEATERS, AND LOTS OF GIRL DOCTORS, POURQUOI PAS?

DURING MY FIRST WEEK OF medical school at the State University of Liege, I found myself studying the anatomy of the entire skeleton. This involved memorizing all the shapes and grooves of every part of the skeleton. Each ridge has a special anatomic name in Latin. My colleagues and I had the unique joy of also learning this in French. In fact, all of our medical courses were taught in French, but as an American planning to return to the United States, we needed to learn in English and Latin. Being in medical school was overwhelming, but I felt like the luckiest man in the world. That being said, I had a lot to absorb during that first week. I tried to spend much time with my Belgian friends to gain in French fluency. Fortunately, I studied quite a bit of French during college, but fluency comes from living in the culture and with the individuals. When I was in medical school in Europe, 50–60% of students were female. At that time in the United States about 10–20% of students were female. Today, it is about a fifty-fifty male-to-female student distribution. This is concerning for such a large country as the United States, because most women are not particularly interested in studying lengthy specialties, such as surgical training, and then moving on to establish a career as a surgeon. A woman finds herself juggling a husband and then working in a very difficult and elite specialty. Certainly, I've had the pleasure of knowing some extremely talented women in neurosurgery, general surgery, cardiac surgery, and orthopedic surgery. I would add to the equation that the vast majority of couples had the husband and wife working as physicians, even if not in the same specialty. Often, children were under the care of a nanny. This is not some template, but it is a common scenario. Knowing that we may be losing many specialties is a serious concern for physicians of my age.

When I was studying in Belgium, we had many Belgian students and a fair number of German, Scandinavian, North African, French, and Middle Eastern students. Belgium is windy and rainy, with some snow in winter. It is not the south of France. The weather was perfect for studying and other indoor sports. Railway tickets were not expensive, so it was easy to travel to Amsterdam or other villages in Holland, Paris, and other French cities. I traveled through many cities over the European continent—not a bad way to live while in your twenties.

MEDICAL SCHOOL, MD (MANY DECEPTIONS)

WHEN I WAS A FIRST-YEAR student, I learned that there was a surgical amphitheater across from the ER. In an amphitheater, students and physicians were able to sit in a glass-enclosed room and view surgery using a video link or studying by looking through the glass enclosure. Although it was difficult to study the surgical details, especially as a first-year student, it was still beyond exciting. When the surgeons came into the OR, the hair on my neck would stand up. I was still planning a career in psychiatry and possibly neurology. I did not see myself as a surgeon.

Each year we placed new textbooks adjacent to the old textbooks from prior years of study. The paradigm was very particular. You studied and learned new material that would then be added to courses already learned to review again. To be competent in medicine, you must have brain circuitry that allows strong if not excellent memory skills. Of course, it demands far more than strong memory skills, but the memory skills are a good start. Depending on your specialty, your life could be far more stressful than that of other specialists—the hours of work, emergency calls, and, if you are a surgeon, concerns about maintaining your skill set and dexterity. We make these decisions about specialties when we are young and have no real idea about consequences. I knew that whatever I chose as a specialist, there was going to be a serious amount of sleep deprivation. This was not an issue in my twenties or thirties. As you get a bit older, though, the notion of sleep takes on a greater importance, especially if you are a surgeon. When I was in medical school, no one ever discussed income. It was of no importance. It is, however, very important because it is a very intimate part of you and your family's lives, if you have a family. Ego, jealousy, fairness, and honesty are all critical issues, and I've seen many private practices or academic departments get quite disabled because of these very same concerns. Some physicians are good entrepreneurs and accountants, but most are not, and it's easy to get lost along the way.

THE WRONG TURN

WHEN I FINALLY GOT TO study psychiatry in medical school, I made two important discoveries, the first being the fascination of studying the textbook. I loved each and every page. The second discovery was when I started working with psychiatrists and patients. Everything changed dramatically for the worst. Translating the texts to the actual clinic work didn't work well for me, personally. It was obfuscated and slow in learning. Psychoanalysis, which is a very important phase of treating mentally ill patients, is very hard to learn and takes way too much time. Pharmacology was not very promising in the 1970s and 1980s. As much as I enjoyed the theory of psychopathology, I couldn't imagine spending my career as a psychiatrist. My next thought was neurology because I seemed to have a strong understanding of the course work. When I worked with patients in the hospital, I felt very comfortable. While I was continuing my clinical work with the residents and other physicians at the hospital, I found that I needed another clinical course, and I chose to take neurology again.

NEUROSURGERY, LIFE BEGINS

THE PROBLEM WAS THAT I had already taken neurology, and there were no longer spots available, so my student counselor advised me to take a course in neurosurgery instead. I thought that it would be interesting to observe, and I thought that most neurologists had seen a fair share of neurosurgery. This turned out to be entirely fallacious; I have never found a neurology resident or trainee working one month, two months, or two hours in neurosurgery. I signed up for the course, and I was surprised that I was the only student in the class. Neurosurgeons were the only specialists interested in spending any functional time in the neurosurgery department. There was the department chief of neurosurgery and four other neurosurgeons working on the staff as senior neurosurgeons, which meant that they had completed their surgical training. There were two resident neurosurgeons. One was in his fourth year of preparation, and the other was in his second year of residency. This was a small but very busy department, and the staff was very well trained. For me now, looking back forty-six years ago, I can say that some of those surgeons were true masters.

My first case to observe was when the chief was planning to treat a burst aneurysm in the brain. An aneurysm is defined as a blister on an artery in the brain. Aneurysms can be found in many locations, sizes, and shapes. If an aneurysm ruptures, about 30–50% of patients don't make it to the hospital. Of those who get to the hospital, successful treatment depends on how impaired the patient is at the onset and the skill set of the surgical team. During most of my career as a neurosurgeon, we treated aneurysms by placing a special metallic clip over the blister so it would not rupture again. This is what we call microsurgery.

There is also another type of treatment that has been going on for over ten years and which is getting better and more sophisticated. This is called endovascular surgery, where the surgeon does not open the head and operate inside the brain. That procedure requires the use of specialized radiologic imaging. The surgeon places special coils inside the arteries of the leg and then the coils are moved through the arteries getting smaller and smaller until the coils are accurately located inside the aneurysm. The coils are then positioned, which should prevent further rupture in the aneurysm. The dynamics of the procedure are very complicated, so we'll let it rest here. It is, however, a very important contribution to aneurysm repair.

In today's world, only a few types of aneurysms are clipped inside the brain. As I was advancing through my schooling, I did have the opportunity to observe other types of general surgery.

Neurosurgery, however, was very different. There was almost absolute silence in the neurosurgery OR—no music and certainly no casual discussion. Absolutely no talking occurred, unless the professor had something to say. There was a large surgical microscope used for microsurgery that made observing easier when you were linked to the video. You had the two surgeons working on the microscope and then other observers watching the video screens. An operating nurse made sure that the surgeons were given the instruments needed at exactly the right time, and then a circulating nurse transferred other needed instrument packs to the surgical staff and the anesthesia staff. The operating microscope and smaller available lights provided an ambiance making visualization easier for those observing surgery. Training to become a master neurosurgeon takes many years of intense practice.

When the surgery started, the professor did everything from start to finish. He opened the scalp with the scalpel. The skull was opened with special bone drills. Underneath the skull, there is an envelope covering the brain, called the dura mater. When the dura mater was opened, we viewed the living brain pulsating with blue veins and red arteries. The color of the brain tissue depended on whether it was healthy or not and to what degree. Whitish, yellow-gray, green, or black were some options. The brain was warm if you had a chance to lightly palpate the organ. Years later, I had great enjoyment allowing an RN or an assistant gently touch the brain to palpate the pulsations. If a tumor was present, allowing one to feel the mass pushing against the brain surface, I promise you will not easily forget how fast your heart was racing.

I stood back in the corner of the OR, absolutely mesmerized. The control, the quiet and the strict attention, was what I needed and wanted. That day, which went very well in the OR, got me thinking quite seriously. I wondered if I was good enough to learn these skills and spend my career working as a neurosurgeon.

Watching this small staff working in this OR changed my life enormously. I had no idea which door I was planning to open.

Earning my MD was a great accomplishment, but then what? It was becoming clearer that I would need to climb a higher mountain if I was chasing neurosurgery. There are three distinct aspects of preparing to pursue neurosurgery. There is the purely cognitive and cerebral segment. This determines if your intellect can absorb and respond to the complex subjects of neuroradiology, neuropathology, and neurosurgery (the mechanics of whether the brain can determine what to do with the information studied by the brain). The second segment is how the brain activates the movements of the hand. This is the hand-eye association. The third segment relies entirely on the dexterity of the hand, fingers, and arms. This is a purely mechanical activity. Without minimizing any aspect of neurosurgery, it is not unlike an accomplished musician, a respected artist, or a highly trained pilot.

The courses required to prepare for a career in neurosurgery were scary and arduous. I studied at Ivy League schools, and I developed a very intense approach. I learned quite a lot of neuroscience in Belgium and elsewhere. I completed my medical studies with honors in my master's degree and my MD. I had numerous options to train for neurosurgery at many institutions, but I stayed where I felt comfortable—in Belgium. There were three residents, or physicians in training, and we were not following each other sequentially. The resident closest to me was two years ahead of me, and the most advanced resident was four years further down the road.

The training in Belgium was more of an apprenticeship than a residency. In the United States, the training was highly maintained, and there were courses and examinations, determining your position in the residency. In Belgium, you needed to learn more independently, which was considerably more difficult.

One day, my professor advised a resident that after four years, he didn't consider him competent enough to continue neurosurgery in Belgium. This very bright young man became a neurologist. It shocked me that a resident could lose his position so easily. At the same time that this was going on with this resident, my professor advised me that to continue in neurosurgery in Belgium, I would have to give up my US citizenship and take on a Belgian passport. My professor was not aware of these consequences, and at this point, I was the only American resident studying in Belgium. I would have to repeat all my neurosurgery in the United States to return there to work. I learned of all this in April, after residencies were planned to start on July 1. I applied for admissions at several institutions and was accepted for the following year, not the coming July.

In the United States, you had to train in general surgery before you started neurosurgery. I would have repeated two years of neurosurgery followed by a year of general surgery before starting my training in neurosurgery in the United States. I was thus going to lose some time, but I decided that I was still young and I'd do what I needed to do to get back to the United States. As far I could see, I was continuing to learn.

FORTUNATELY, NOT TOO LATE

ONE NIGHT I RECEIVED A phone call from the professor of neurosurgery at the University of Miami-Jackson Memorial Hospital. This was in May, and I was told that their department was interested in accepting me as an additional resident, which meant that I would start general surgery in July and my neurosurgery training the following July. Most universities accept one or two residents into training. In Miami, they were willing to accept three residents. My professor from Miami knew our university in Liege, Belgium, as an illustrious university on the European continent. He also liked that I was fluent in French and my grades in medical school were good. He decided to accept me earlier, if I was still interested in coming. I told him that the luggage would be packed that evening. University of Miami-Jackson Memorial Hospital was considered one of the largest and most prestigious trauma centers in the United States.

I learned quite a bit, studying in Belgium. I prepared medicine at a great university and strengthened my brain "smarts" to keep me moving forward. I loved learning another language and met some fascinating students from all over Europe and elsewhere.

I found my career because of a small group of physicians who hypnotized me. Moving forward, my heart dreamed I would learn to be as talented.

JACKSON MEMORIAL HOSPITAL, INSOMNIA, DIRE STRAIT, AND WORK OF LIFE

IN TWO WEEKS, I WAS living in Miami, getting ready to start my residency. The hospital was magnificent, and after moving from the chilly, rainy, and gray Belgian city streets of Western Europe, I found myself wearing surgical green scrub suits, white clogs, and a long lab coat as I attempted to monitor my way through the many corridors of Jackson Memorial Hospital (JMH). Of course, at that time I didn't realize that all my free time cruising around my subtropical climate could be caught on one hand. At JMH, your work stopped after you were told it was time to go home—and not a second sooner.

Only the chief resident can make that happen, and this is a much-cherished position. In today's world, the residents are very restricted with the number of hours worked. When I was a resident, work started at 5:00 a.m. and lasted until the chief resident was disposed to close "shop." At the end of the workday, the evening emergency staff on call started the evening and night hours, and only a junior resident and a senior resident were available. The chief resident did not return to the hospital at night unless there was a phenomenal crisis.

We often worked over a hundred hours a week. No one complained, because we felt that any cases we didn't care for were cases lost. Residents were completely and fully awake, awake, somewhat awake, alert, thinking about it, considering it, somewhat thoughtful, drowsy, sleepy, and 911.

INSOMNIA

IT WAS NOT UNCOMMON TO park my car in the early morning in some corner of a massive parking garage, forget where I parked because I'd lost my parking stub, and spent two hours looking for my vehicle after having worked thirty-six hours without sleep. This, of course, was only one part of the adventure. Driving home was the second part of this installment. Somehow, I would find my car and drive over an hour to my condo, shower, and get to bed to awaken cold and in a sweat, realizing I had no idea how I made it home.

My year in general surgery truly prepared me for working nonstop. I learned how to take care of patients in the ICU, both adults and neonates, and by the end of the year, I felt ready to handle many critical problems. Even though I was planning to specialize in neurosurgery, there were many opportunities to operate, and I performed several appendectomies, cholecystectomies, and several hernias.

For two months, I worked in the cardiothoracic program. The chief loved me there and tried to get me to stay in general surgery and then specialize in cardiac surgery. I enjoyed it, and I was allowed to do some cases that I was probably a little young for (with an appropriate assistant at my side), and as Jackson Memorial Hospital was one of the busiest trauma centers in the country, the residents were constantly learning and working. I seem to love so much of medicine, but I knew that neurosurgery was where I aimed my arrow. It was a wonderful year for me, and I was grateful for the opportunity and all that I had learned.

WALK OF LIFE

TRAINING IN NEUROSURGERY MEANT YOU needed to become a master in neuroanatomy, neurophysiology, neuropharmacology, neuropathology, clinical neurosurgery, neuroradiology, neurology, and critical intensive care. I would also add that we were expected to care for anyone from the neonates (infants) to beyond ninety years old. When I was training in neurosurgery, the program lasted seven years. It felt like we were ready for our social security payments when we completed our studies. We also needed to have a research thesis. Our professors were very interested in training for academic careers, which meant working at a university hospital, continuing research, and teaching.

To graduate from your training program, the faculty needed to approve, and you needed to be successful in Phase I of the board-certification examination. This is a written examination. Phase II is given at a minimum of three years after the completion of residency, but it could be four or five years, depending on how many physicians wanted to take the examination and where you found yourself on the guest list. Most residents complete Phase I during their chief-residency year. Not everyone gets chosen as chief resident. Our chief of the department made us take the written examination starting in our second year of residency, but it was used as a teaching examination. The faculty wanted to be sure that the residents were studying and not just sleeping when not running around the hospital.

When I trained in residency, we were expected to handle most every problem involving the brain and/or spine, at all ages. As the cliché goes, the buck stops here! The truth was that we were not ready to handle any problem at any time. Working in neurosurgery, I learned very quickly that there was much to learn, and it seemed impossible to get to the final page of the last book. Polishing your surgical skills started the first day you ask for a scalpel and ended when you returned it for that last time.

There are so many specialties within the overall "world" of neurosurgery that seven years are not long enough. This created fellowship programs. After you have completed your residency, you can study for one or two years at a very specialized university. This will allow you the opportunity to become subspecialized in areas like pediatric neurosurgery, cerebrovascular and endovascular surgery, functional surgery for patients with Parkinson's and other diseases as well as epilepsy, neuro-oncology surgery for very complicated tumors of the brain and spine surgery, which is a very common fellowship. Years ago, most physicians who went into fellowships were planning on studying and working in academic surgery. This is not entirely true today, and many study fellowships but still work in private practice and not at the university. This is particularly true of pediatric and spine surgery.

I've met brilliant students, residents, and neurosurgeons, and common polling suggests that neurosurgeons are the second-most-common desirable job after president of the United States. Rocket science is a close third. As usual, it's because people do not know what lies behind that famous closed door. Some surgeons may struggle more dramatically than others may. It is, however, clear that the trajectory is not a simple one. If you somehow believed that you were born to pass from the womb to brain surgeon, there are going to be some bad days ahead. You will find yourself staring at your own reflection and trying determinedly to see past your swollen and blurry eyes as some impossibly complicated question comes your way at 3:00 a.m.

Training as a surgeon requires an element of egotism, jealousy, and envy. There will always be those smarter, more dexterous, and more creative. The sooner you realize this, the better your life will be.

You need to define yourself and determine why you are doing this for a living. There is much to lose during this adventure, and you must be ready for those losses. We can learn to deal with success and wonderful results as a neurosurgeon. How do we deal with patients dying? How do we deal with a disability affecting one of our patients? If you are competent, you will have families and friends loving you and always on your sides. However, no matter how experienced and competent you are, you will always find some against you, for one reason or another. My experience is that the love runs deeper.

We don't learn how to deal with these very real emotions during college, medical school, or your career. Life changes as we age, as do our emotions and maturity. As a young physician, I created a certain image of how I should appear as a neurosurgeon.

My intellectual and physical aptitudes were of great concern. My attitudes, responses, and reactions changed remarkably as I matured.

For me, personally, I encountered two real differences emotively. As a younger man, I didn't cry. When patients died or were harmed and I was involved in the care, I studied constantly and learned everything I could to avoid a bad response in the future. My attention was very mechanical and directed. As years passed, I became more intent regarding my capabilities as a specialist. Most people believe that neurosurgeons are brilliant, have ice water in their blood, are unemotional, have no fear, and shed no tears. The better I became as a specialist and the older I grew, the more I cried for good results and sadness. And cry I did!

During my training in neurosurgery, I found, as expected, that some specialty work was more interesting and exciting than others were. For me, I found a real interest in pediatric surgery and cerebrovascular surgery. These fellowships did not exist when I was specializing, so I became a general neurosurgeon, with a subspecialty interest in caring for infants, babies, and children, as well as caring for patients with AVM (arteriovenous malformations) and aneurysms.

After twenty-nine years of working as a neurosurgeon, I went to sleep with a smile or not. This is the nature of the fluidity of this work. When I placed my scalpel down for the last time, even though I was unaware of this reality, I was thoroughly and entirely convinced that I was still training and polishing and just getting better. I have seen residents and completely certified surgeons quit for various reasons but obviously very dramatic life changes. Are you the tortoise or the hare? How do we trial one against the other?

When I was getting toward the end of my training, I had developed a clear interest in pediatric neurosurgery, and so I was able to perform a lot of extra work with neurologically afflicted children. The year before I became the chief resident in neurosurgery, I performed very well on Phase I of the board certification examination. This meant that I could spend the entire chief resident year operating where I was most interested and not worry about preparing for any exams. At that time, I encountered two formidable cases.

DIRE STRAIT

One morning, I received a phone call from a pediatric intensivist (intensive care unit specialist from the pediatric age group) working at a remote hospital. A woman in her last term of gestation was shot in the abdomen with a handgun, releasing a .45-caliber projectile through the uterus into the cranium of the fetus. The projectile penetrated deep into the brain. An emergency cesarean section was performed, and both the mother and the fetus survived.

The injury occurred seven weeks before the phone call to me. Initially, everyone expected the baby to die, but he survived, and ultimately the baby was removed from his respirator. He also started to feed normally. The only issue was that when the baby was held up, if his head was lying down on the right-hand side, the left arm and leg would become paralyzed. If the head was turned toward the left-hand side, the right leg and arm would stop moving. When the head was in a neutral position, both arms and legs started moving spontaneously and with normal strength.

The baby had already had a new CAT scan (CT) performed, which demonstrated a large projectile (bullet) floating in a large cyst deep within the brain. When the head moved, the projectile would move within the cyst and then strike the brain tissue adjacent to the cyst cavity. This would cause the injury to the opposite arm and leg. Clearly, this had never been seen or described in medical history.

We immediately transferred the baby and his mother to the intensive care unit at JMH. We prepared to bring the baby for surgery later that day. My professor advised me that I would perform the surgery. I had studied all the X-rays and discussed the surgery with the baby's mother. I explained the risks and complications and that we all believed that removing the bullet from the brain could avoid permanent injury. The skull at the age of seven weeks is extremely thin, and we placed a neuro ultrason, which is a special type of imaging device, to see beneath the superficial structures of the skull and brain. With the ultrason in position, I saw exactly where the projectile was engaged within the brain. The infant was placed under general anesthesia, and the surgeons positioned the sterile drapes.

I placed a small incision in the scalp at my desired target. The very thin skull was opened using small operating scissors. The dura mater (the envelope over the brain) was opened, and I then made a small incision in the brain, overlying the site where the projectile entered the brain itself. With the operating microscope, I magnified the cyst and found the projectile immediately. I introduced a small forceps and gently removed the entire bullet. There was no bleeding, and it appeared that everything went very well. I had to give the projectile to the sheriff's department, some of whom were present in the OR to retrieve the bullet. I'm more than certain that the sheriff never forgot that surgery. I know for sure that I didn't!

This would have been on cable news today. The child and mother did perfectly well. *Life* magazine wanted to have a special section, but the baby's mother refused. I did write a publication for a well-known medical neurosurgery journal, and I got a little "famous" for a short period. I received letters and questions from neurosurgeons living and working all over the world. The piece was printed in a newspaper in Germany and was printed in the *New York Times*. It was very exciting for the entire department. Over the years, I was offered the chance to lecture many groups about brain trauma. The first photograph on the screen was always a very large bullet sitting in the middle of a baby's skull. This was always joined by many oohs and aahs.

DIRE STRAIT II

ANOTHER CASE INVOLVED A YOUNG child of six, presenting with a rare case of a tumor in the pituitary gland. The pituitary gland is considered the "master gland" of the brain and is mostly responsible for transporting and channeling the most important hormones in the brain. The pituitary gland is attached to a stalk underneath the base of the brain, in a bony saddle between the eye sockets. Several problems can occur with the pituitary gland, such as a tumor that could cause an excess of one or more hormones, leading to problems with physical appearance, blood pressure, growth, metabolism, thyroid function, premature puberty, and various other medical issues and symptoms. The more common problem is a tumor in the pituitary gland that grows without causing any additional formation of hormone. Usually, the tumor would compress the pituitary gland by growing larger, and that could lead to failure in the function of the pituitary. Any of these tumors can grow and cause compression on the surrounding brain. In the case of the brain, near the pituitary gland, the nerves controlling eyesight are immediately next to the gland, and when a tumor grows slightly above one centimeter, it could affect vision. Many patients presenting with pituitary tumors do need surgery. This, of course, is not in every case, but it is common. Some tumors can be treated with medications and radiation.

In this particular case, the tumor was liberating too much cortisone from the pituitary gland. This caused problems with her stature, exceptional acne, high blood pressure, and early puberty. Her vision was normal, so the tumor size was very small and what we call a microadenoma, or smaller than one centimeter (cm). This tumor had a medical name—Cushing's disease. The diagnosis was made by examination of the child, special blood tests, and imaging with special scanning. A hormone specialist called an endocrinologist made the diagnosis, and the patient was then transferred to neurosurgery. At this time, I was the chief resident and was very excited to be caring for this patient.

The most common way to operate on this patient was entering through the mouth and nostril or just through the nostril. In situations when the tumor is very large or has an unusual appearance, like an hourglass shape, we open the skull (craniotomy) and remove the tumor from above. Either way, the surgery will be done using a surgical operating microscope. In this case, we operated through the mouth and nostril, and we removed the microadenoma from the pituitary gland. It was determined that this patient was the youngest with Cushing's disease.

I wrote another manuscript for a neurosurgical journal that included a photograph showing that her physical appearance was entirely normal.

Shortly after this paper was written, I was invited to prepare my presentation to the American Association of Neurosurgery-

Pediatric Division. At this meeting were some of the most well-known pediatric neurosurgeons in the world. I was now a resident who had written two papers never described before, and I was getting some attention. At this time, I was considering studying pediatric neurosurgery, and I was invited to join many different universities. That was all very seductive.

Of course, there is that saying that we plan, and God laughs. I spent some serious time thinking about my decisions. I came to realize that I was not a research person, and research was something you must do if you wanted to work in academics. Most surgeons worked at one university and then another as they climbed the academic ladder. I enjoyed lecturing and teaching, but my love was the OR. As a pediatric neurosurgeon, I would have been working on children and would not have gotten a chance to work on other problems, such as brain aneurysms. I made my decision, and now I planned to complete my residency and look around for a private practice job.

One day in October 1985, I was treating a patient with a ruptured aneurysm in the brain. The chief of the department was watching me work while he was in the assistant's spot. This was very common for me at that stage in the game. Fortunately, everything went well, and I identified the burst aneurysm and placed an aneurysm clip on the injured artery. This was a life-and-death situation. Because of my interests in aneurysms, I managed to treat a fair number of these problems while I was finishing my residency and many times after my residency was completed. This patient was in his early forties. When we closed his head and the bandages were placed, the anesthesia was slowly reversed, and the patient woke up immediately. He left the hospital without a hitch.

After the surgery was completed that day in October, I left the OR and stepped into the corridor between the various ORs at the university hospital. My professor told me that he wanted to talk to me in the hallway. He had already told me it was a great case, and I figured that as I was the chief resident, my chief of the department needed me to take care of a problem. The rule was that we had really bad problems, bad problems, problems, or little problems.

My chief approached me and advised me that he had a little surprise for me. I was going to be graduated six months early. This was great, except for the fact that it meant in two months. I barely had time to sit down and write the surgery plan for the next day. As chief resident, my responsibilities were to schedule all the surgeries, emergency or not, to go on rounds (seeing all of the patients in the entire department), to arrange for lectures, to discuss any of the problems with the professors, and somehow to operate on about ten very complex cases each week. Clearly, there were other duties, but while writing this story, I determined I was working thirty-two hours/day, so I may have overestimated how important I thought myself.

CENTRAL FLORIDA
AND OPENING THE DOORS

ONE OF THE OTHER PROFESSORS in neurosurgery told me of a good group near Orlando. When they found out I wasn't going into pediatrics, they called me and invited me to meet them. I had someone cover me for the weekend (as the chief resident, I was always on call), and I took a plane to Orlando where I met someone and was driven by limousine to central Florida.

The medical clinic was quite beautiful, and I was very impressed. One of the surgeons was retiring, and so there were two fully working surgeons, and I would be the third. The hospital had all the important paraphernalia. I was taken to dinner, and I guess I was drunk enough, because the following week, they sent me a contract to sign, which I did.

Every graduation time, either one or two chief residents had to say good-byes to the entire department. I was the only chief resident, and it was Christmas time. As expected, I had to listen to a roaring roast on my behalf, but when it came to the good-byes, it was a different deal. My chief of the department told me I was the best resident he had ever taught (which had something to do with what was in his glass at the time) and how I would be missed. My younger residents were happy to drive me to near Orlando. I reminded how my chief professor went out for me and gave me a shot at the position after they had already hired two residents. I was the third resident and unexpected. One of those residents dropped out after two years. My life had changed so dramatically in Miami. I truly thanked everyone, and a lot of tears were mixed with all the Christmas presents.

TAKE ME OUT TO THE BALLGAME

I STARTED TO WORK IN early January 1986 becoming an independent neurosurgeon. The most important part of that day is that I met my wife without either of us being aware.

One day on a very hot and sunny afternoon, a group of young, strong, and athletic people were playing softball. A twenty-two-year-old young man was struck quite hard in the head, and he apparently fell to the ground unconscious. He was transferred to the hospital in a coma, and a CT scan of the brain revealed bruising of the brain and edema (swelling). He was quite ill and was not responding well. One of my associates was responsible for his care because he was on call at the time of the injury. For one week, this young man remained in a coma and was worsening.

At the end of the call week, I was on call starting Friday evening. Later that night, about 1:00 a.m., I got a phone call from the ICU nurse, and I was told that the patient appeared to be brain-dead. I had never met this patient, but I was aware of his terrible condition. He had developed extreme swelling within the brain, and not all his reflexes were working. He was treated with all the various medications for brain swelling and seizures.

He had a special monitor, known as an intracranial pressure device, placed within the brain to calibrate the degree of pressure in the brain. His injuries were on both sides of the brain, but mostly the right. My associate did not expect him to survive.

I drove to the hospital and met the patient. Examining the patient I agreed that he appeared clinically brain-dead. He had not yet had an EEG, but based on everything else available, including his heart rate slowing down and a loss of all his reflexes, I believed we would lose him. I then met the patient's mother, who clearly was the "boss." The patient's wife didn't say a word. They had a little baby girl sleeping on her mother's lap. I told them the situation and advised the patient's mother and his wife that survival was not expected. The patient's mother looked at me and then said that if there was anything I could do, even if it meant he would survive alive in a vegetative state, she would visit him every day of her life. I told her that we make our decisions based on the examinations and tests and following the current state of affairs, I could offer one particular option. The chance of his returning was still close to zero. My option was to radically remove all the swollen and dead brain while hoping that the healthier residual brain tissue might reduce the existing high pressure in the brain.

We didn't have much time to discuss options and concerns. The patient's mother took my hands, and she prayed. Her eyes were tearing fully, and I had my work waiting for me. He was in a deep coma and not responding. His pupillary reflexes were not working nor were his corneal reflexes. These tests determine if the most critical circuitry in the brain was active. His heart rate was very slow, and his blood pressure was very erratic, jumping up and down. He was dying!

I opened his skull very quickly, and then we opened the dura mater around the brain on the right side, which was the most severely injured. I incised a very large opening of the envelope and beneath we could see that the brain was discolored and abnormal, cold and not pulsating. I then started to resect as much of the sick, swollen brain as I could identify. When the brain is swollen so dramatically, it's very difficult to identify and determine the anatomy and structures of the motor circuits, the emotional circuitry, and the issues assisting memory and the other "higher" functions for ideas, creativity, and logic. The injury was on the right side, and the swelling was extended toward the left and worsening. I continued to work, and ultimately, I resected an excessive amount of sick and swollen brain. This was called a right frontal lobectomy. With most of the brain removal completed, I brought in the operating microscope, to be particularly cautious with the very deep areas of the brain.

When I was completed, the brain was palpating, and the swelling was dramatically improved. The surgery lasted over five hours in the OR. His heart rate was now normal, and I was beginning to believe that the patient had some chance for some form of survival.

I went back to the family and explained that it was now on the "wings of the angels." I'm not sure when that phrase became a part of me, but it is part of my spirit.

One week later, the reflexes in his eyes were normal, and a week after that we were able to get the ventilator respirator removed. Two weeks later, he started to speak and was moving his arms and legs. This was phenomenal, but the best was yet to come. He went off to a good rehabilitation where he stayed for several more weeks.

After several months, he was on a television show that I never saw, but I was told he appeared quite normal. His only issue was some amnesia, but he was improving with time. I saw him about sixteen months later at my office. His rehabilitation was performed out of the state of Florida, so it took a while for me to see him again. I examined him and could not find anything wrong. His walking, balance, coordination, strength, speech, and now driving and working appeared entirely normal. This did not include a neuropsychology examination, but I read that other studies suggested minor memory issues. He returned to his original job.

WHEN BENIGN IS NOT GOOD

THAT DAY WAS INTERESTING, BECAUSE of all the good things, he had not the slightest idea of who I was. Over the years, I had many of these: "I do not remember you, Doctor." I have no complaints regarding these forms of amnesia. As an example, years ago I was traveling with my family as we were awaiting the arrival of a passenger plane at a regional airport. We had six people talking at the same time, which was clearly our modus operandi. Another family noticed us and approached us. One of the gentlemen in his group introduced himself and the others traveling with him.

It turned out that, several years before this chance encounter, I had been asked to care for this gentleman's mother, who had been quite ill, with a very large and benign brain tumor called a meningioma. The tumor had been attached underneath the brain and to the base of the skull and many important, complex structures. She'd been seventy-eight years old and very disabled. Some of her family had heard of me, as a neurosurgeon, and I had been highly recommended to care for this patient. I'd made it very clear that the tumor, although benign (not malignant), had been growing for many years and had tunneled around arteries, veins, nerves, and many other webs, rendering this surgery almost inoperable. One of the family had spoken with a neurosurgeon at another university, and after reviewing the MRI (magnetic resonance imaging), he'd told them she would not survive or would perform very poorly. He would not perform the surgery, and I had agreed with him.

I'd then found myself in a situation I'd seen before, on many occasions. This patient had been gravely ill, and the choice had been transferring her to hospice (a noninvasive form of nursing) or pursuing surgery. The patient had made it clear that hospice had not been an option. We'd talked for many hours, and we'd prayed. We had pursued surgery, and I had operated for eleven hours. She had been recovering, and I had started to look for the "wings on angels," but after three days, she had sustained a massive stroke that had led to her passing.

Why the story? My involvement with this patient and her family had occurred several years prior, but they recognized me at the airport and felt the need to hug my shoulders and thank me for everything I'd done for them. Over the years, many patients forgot the face or name, but it all traveled through my heart and that I never forgot.

Back to the story of my young patient, his aunt was there, and she wrote a poem that she placed on my desk. My wife and I were awaiting the arrival of our first child. The patient's aunt knew we were waiting for a son. She wrote in her poem, "Thanks for giving us two new sons back." Of course, there was much more written, but it has sat on the top of my bookcase since 1991.

I've been very aggressive as a surgeon over my career, but this particular case changed me. I believe that a very high percentage of patients, like this last one, would have died because no one tried. Every now and then, the "wings on angels" sit on someone's shoulder in the OR. I never figured out how to find them, but Lord knows, I kept looking.

A TRUE MEDUSA

ONE DAY, A YOUNG MAN was waterskiing behind a powerful ski boat. He was thirty-six years old at the time and visiting Florida for some holiday. This young man lived in Switzerland and worked as a percussionist in the symphony orchestra. He was a masterful skier on alpine mountains and was thus a very athletic individual. One day he got on the speedboat following a lengthy waterski run. He seemed alert but confused, and he was having difficulty speaking English and German, his two fluent languages.

The patient had problems with simple calculations and confusing his right and left. He had issues with reading and writing, and it is important to note that he was right handed. This suggested that the left side of the brain was the dominant circuitry for speech dynamics, including writing, speaking, and understanding. Part of the left side of the brain determines understanding the difference between the right and left side and calculations, whether simple or complex. It's easy to imagine, or maybe not, that every structure in the brain has some bizarre name associated with it, such as Broca's and Wernicke's areas, and the angular and supramarginal gyri. It's probably a good idea to stay away from the fancy stuff!

His balance, strength, and coordination appeared to be normal. He was sent to radiology for a computerized tomographic scan (CT), and this revealed a significantly sized blood clot on the left side of the brain. The location of the blood clot explained his neurologic impairment. For someone his age, we had to consider this diagnosis to be called an arteriovenous malformation. Normally, arteries transport oxygenated blood to the capillaries and then the veins, which are low in oxygen, before getting new oxygenation at the heart and lungs. Arteries are red, and veins are blue. In this illness, also called AVM, there are no capillaries and the arteries connect to the veins in an abnormal type of mapping. The connection is fragile and friable, and it can burst open, causing bleeding in the brain tissue.

We sent the patient to be scheduled for an angiogram, which allowed the radiologists to administer a special dye into the arteries. That dye would travel into the abnormal AVM. When the blood clot is large enough to cause significant impairment into the brain, the neurosurgeon's task is to remove the clot and disconnect the abnormal connection, also called a nidus, from the arteries and veins. Aneurysms and AVMs are clearly the most complex brain surgeries to be performed. If I had to guess between the two, I'd say that the AVM is the greatest nightmare. The angiogram identified the AVM as we expected, and the decision was to go to the OR. Given his athleticism and his skill set as a symphony musician, he had much to lose.

The brain, when exposed, was swollen and bulging beyond the opened skull. There were numerous areas of hemorrhage on the surface of the brain substance, and this was expanding deep within the cavities of the brain. We then studied the architecture of the AVM, which meant identifying the fragile arteries interposing with the nidus. These structures needed to be seen in a 3-D configuration, which was complex since the geometry of the malformation had to be dissected one micron at a time. The veins involved in the AVM were no longer blue, as they should have been, but were red since the oxygenated blood from the arteries passed through the poorly functional nidus and did not enter the substance of the brain tissue. This meant the brain was deficient of oxygen and was thus involved in a form of stroke.

The veins were massively engorged because the pressure within the arteries was transferred into the veins. If our blood pressure is 180/60, in an AVM the 180 transmits to the veins, which causes the engorgement and fragility. Normally, the capillary bed caused a reduction in the pressure from the arteries to the veins, as the normal and functional oxygenated blood cells transferred to the brain tissue. Now, we had a fragile spider web of arteries, a nidus, and engorged red veins. The pressure within the AVM was not like the normal pressure in an artery, and so a rupture of the nidus did not attempt exsanguination, as was often the case in a true aneurysm rupture. An AVM can become symptomatic by a seizure, stroke, or, finally, hemorrhage. Of course, the "coup de grace" (final cause of death) would be a combination of all three possibilities. Some people have aneurysms or AVMs that never cause symptoms and are not diagnosed throughout the length of an otherwise normal lifestyle. That would be a good definition of lucky. These prior paragraphs explain why I never slept well before operating if it wasn't an emergency surgery.

The surgery involved microsurgery with the operating microscope and lasted many hours. It was extremely important not to obliterate any of the engorged emptying veins because that would have caused a certain elevation of the pressure within the nidus, potentially leading to a catastrophe.

In this case, we were able to carefully aspirate the blood clots and identify the appropriate attachments to the arteries, connecting to the almost miniscule penetrating blood vessels, creating the very complicated nidus. We then had to resect all of these channels until the only corridors available were the residual veins, which were now of a normal size and color since the AVM was exenterated.

Watching the veins change to blue was always like reaching the summit of Everest. If any portion of the surgery became problematic, the patient could have a massive stroke or die from a dramatic hemorrhage. It took a lot of teaching and assisting, over years, to get to a point that a surgeon could perform these procedures and be ready to troubleshoot all the hidden traps.

This patient did remarkably well following his surgery and began his course of rehabilitation, lasting about three weeks. He was then transported to Switzerland to continue with his recovery. About one year after his adventure started, I received a large business envelope at my office, addressed from Switzerland. Within the envelope, was a personalized letter to me, a copy of a newspaper article discussing his illness, and most importantly, a photograph of my patient performing again with the symphony orchestra. I wrote him a letter back with an updated photograph, and once again, I found those "wings."

FRIENDS, ROMANS, AND COUNTRYMEN

I WORKED FOR SEVERAL YEARS in central Florida, and as this was the start of my rookie year, it was an important part of my life. I learned a lot of medicine from my associates, but mostly spinal surgery. My training in Miami was strongly intensified upon my career as a cranial surgeon. I was able to perform a lot of the more complex cranial cases coming into our clinic because I had the interest and wanted to polish those skills as best possible. I learned a lot of the tricks needed for spine surgery, and this came almost entirely from working with my associates at the early stages of my career.

I was now married, with two children, and my understanding of entrepreneurship, which was originally zero, started to develop. I became a bookkeeper, as it was viable to know, entirely, where the dollars and cents were located. When we spend so many years studying and training, we don't pay attention to the fiducial dynamics. I've heard this time and time again. Get help to understand your employment agreements; they can ruin a department. We want to be doctors first and foremost, but we also need to function as businesspeople.

When I started working, the clinic had partnerships,

including neurologists and neurosurgeons. These partners received the same base salary and then split the bonuses at the end of the fiscal year. This meant that the partners, both neurologists and neurosurgeons, earned the same exact income, despite the differences in the levels of our production, or vacation time. I was not aware of this fiscal structure when I signed up. I was given a very nice salary, but I was told that I would have to work five years before becoming a partner. After two years of working, I became curious and asked the clinic manager to explain the accounting to me. The manager had to get permission for me to study the accounting, but ultimately it came my way. I became aware that my production levels were higher, by far, than any other physician at the clinic. I was, as I already knew, taking far less vacation time. The two busiest neurosurgeons were not yet partners, and we were producing far more income than the other physicians who were already partners. I found out that neurologists usually did not earn what neurosurgeons earn while working in the same clinic. This was extremely rare. Remembering Miami, when I applied for a job, I looked at one clinic because I had so little time to study options. My base salary was very generous, but I never studied any of the bookkeeping.

After two years, I had a discussion with my other nonpartner associate, and we met with the partners of the clinic. I suggested that we restructure the accounting paradigm and that we all receive the same base salary, as this had been going on for some time, but the final bonus would be partitioned based upon the final production income. My associate and I agreed that we become partners immediately. Our CPA developed an equation to distribute the final bonus at the end of the fiscal year. Every year, I earned the highest income because of the work done, and I took far less vacation than other physicians did. As everyone was getting the same initial base salary, any physician could potentially increase his final production bonus by taking less vacation time and increasing production income at the clinic and in the hospital. Vacation time was a minimum of six weeks but could be well beyond, which was usual.

The changes were immediate, as they didn't want to lose the two highest producers, but it created significant problems. I was the youngest and getting paid the most each year. At first, I was "chastised" that I didn't have any children at the time, and so I didn't need as much income. One of the partners disagreed with my theological attachments, although an apology was eventually forthcoming. Other physicians forgot they could earn as much if they worked as hard and as long. Obviously, it was very difficult for a neurologist to produce the same income as a surgeon, although certainly not impossible. Neurologists can earn similar incomes to neurosurgeons if they own the clinic and all of the accessories and testing devices within. Neurologists can earn infusion systems and, more importantly, CT scans and MRI scan. There are EEG and sleep disorder clinics and many other options. You need to earn the devices to eventually create the significant returns. This, of course, involves capitalizing quite significantly. The CPA created the distribution income for the final bonus, and everyone was in full agreement. This was very difficult for me, because despite accepting a very uncommon accounting plan, I, once again, did not feel good in my "own skin." After about seven years, the goodwill was dissipating, and I was no longer enjoying my work. When it came to income, I was concerned about fairness, honesty, and morality. This, unfortunately, is not the rule everywhere you turn.

I thus learned something about business, including envy, jealousy, ego, and a degree of distrust. I didn't like that part of it, and ultimately I became interested in searching for other opportunities. As a Jedi Master would say, "The door open, say I."

WISCONSIN AND FOUR SEASONS

ULTIMATELY, MY CAREER CONTINUED, AND I joined a multispecialty clinic in central Wisconsin. I was there for over twenty years. I was associated with some very talented specialists, and I found myself working, as usual, in the midst of some very incredible adventures. It was common to have neurosurgical cases sent by helicopter to our hospital and, if the weather permitted, from northern Wisconsin, Minnesota, and Michigan.

When my wife and our young children, decided to move to Wisconsin, I had to find a map to see exactly where we were heading. GPS (global positioning system) was not yet on my dashboard. We were looking for a "Norman Rockwell-esque" theme, with four seasons for our children and to grow up in, with snow in the winter. After living here for over twenty years, I promise that in my family, we had seen enough snow for a while. When I became a neurosurgeon, I was certain that I would need to move to an urban center. My belief was that neurosurgery was performed in large medical centers, which would not be possible in rural or semirural regions.

RUDOLPH THE RED-NOSED REINDEER(S)

CARDIAC MEDICINE AND NEUROSCIENCES BECAME very prosperous for most hospitals. I was very happy to find neurosurgery at a trauma center across the street from a cornfield. Not very Norman Rockwell, but it worked well for us. Driving around was easy, except for one particular issue. In the Midwest, we call them deer. You may have heard of them. I know I've written about an occasional medical journal or two, but in Wisconsin, I had two deer hit two of my cars in almost exactly twenty-four hours apart. One jumped out of the woods on the driver side at 5:15 a.m., and almost twenty-four hours later, a second assailed us on the empty passenger side at 5:30 a.m.

I called the phone, and, of course, a young, pretty blonde with a leather holster, shining gun, and spiffy badge showed up. Despite my trembling, I acted as if this was an everyday event. The truth was that the deer excrement was easily mixed with an artful contribution provided by the neurosurgeon driving. Unfortunately, both attempts at resuscitation failed, so I looked carefully, but no "wings" were found.

THE SOUND OF MUSIC

ONE OF MY FIRST CASES involved a ten-year-old boy who became sick with headaches and vomiting, and he had gait and balance disturbance. He was studied by his pediatrician, and a CT scan of the brain was performed, followed by an MRI (magnetic resonance imaging).

He was then sent to my office, and it appeared to me that he had a benign brain tumor in the back of the brain (the cerebellum). The tumor had all the signals of a juvenile astrocytoma. I examined him and explained everything I knew about the probable diagnosis. I explained that if we got the entire tumor out, then this would be considered curable. I discussed how the surgery was performed and that whether benign or malignant, brain surgery was already a somewhat dangerous enterprise. Malignant was always one of those "massive ghosts," but I felt our diagnosis was a good one. One issue that was always extremely important was that patients and families could choose to go elsewhere for care unless the situation was a medical emergency. In this case, as in the vast majority of others, the family decided to keep the patient with us.

He was hospitalized shortly after his diagnosis was suggested, and he was admitted to the hospital for surgery. For this operation, the patient was positioned as if he or she was lying on a park bench. In a park bench position, the patient was almost completely face down, with the head turned enough to get to the very back of the skull and upper back portion of the neck. It was an awkward position but commonly used. Special computerized imaging called stereotaxis allowed the surgeon and physician assistant to guide the trajectory of the scalp incision and bone removal and determine the incision of the brain to help decide the corridor to the tumor mass. With microsurgery and ultrason, we were able to visualize the geometry of the tumor and the depth from the surface of the brain. We were able to remove what I felt was all of the mass, and it was determined to be benign. It was felt to be curable.

During one of his visits to my office, the patient and his family asked about football. I explained that to do the surgery, we needed to remove a small segment of the skull, and I felt that hard impact athletics was not a great idea. I said it was perhaps a better idea to get him interested in music and learn an instrument, as something a little safer for him and possibly a lot of fun.

Several years later, my wife and some of our children were watching a concert in the high school auditorium, and when it was over, a nice woman approached me and asked me to look at the stage at one of the saxophonists. It turned out to be her son, and he'd become quite a talented musician. I would like to say that I advised him to choose the saxophone when he was ten years old, but that would be a minor fantasy. The truth was that she hugged me and began crying as she thanked me for saving her son's life and guided him along his way through life. He was offered a full scholarship to music college, and shortly after our talk, a newscaster came to my office to discuss his story for the local television. My being approached, by patients and their families in front of my own family, happened many times—in front of restaurants, theaters, airports, and stores. I was proud in front of my children, but I always worried about setting the bar too high. Whatever they chose, my wife and I were supportive and set no expectations or exceptions.

I've been on television a few times. When I was a chief resident in Miami, I was part of a surgical team caring for a young high school football player who had broken his neck and paralyzed his spinal cord. For some reason, the newscaster asked me about the injury and the surgery when I was the chief resident. The other issue was that the father of the patient was a retired professional football player in the NFL Hall of Fame and an attorney. One of my professors did have something to say to the patient's father later. The father said he had planned to do everything in his power to help his son's life and anyone else afflicted by this trauma. My professor told him if he could create and pursue various tributes and multimedia productions, he would earn many millions of dollars for the university, and it would help to make a difference. That discussion led to the Miami Cure for Paralysis. This is now the most famous clinical and research system in the world. The young man earned a PhD in psychology, and his life became enormously fulfilled from a terrible tragedy. For me, I was there for the first video and photographs, and I listened to the initial discussions leading to the Miami Cure for Paralysis. At the time, I didn't want anything to do with newscasters, and I just wanted to go hide!

DOWN BY THE RIVER, I SHOT MY BABY

ANOTHER SITUATION INVOLVED A YOUNG girl of eleven living at home with her family. A man living at a halfway house nearby came into the child's home, carrying a gun, and he decided to shoot everyone in the family. Two people, including the eleven-year-old girl, were shot in the head. The neurosurgeon on call was another associate, and he called me, asking for some help. I decided to take the younger girl to the OR as she was dying. This injury involved the back of the brain and was catastrophic. We were able to stop the hemorrhaging and remove the projectiles, but the brain was injured in a very critical area, and she developed a condition called malignant pulmonary edema. Normally, in pulmonary edema, the lung is full of fluid because of heart failure. This edema is more critical and does not respond like typical heart failure. The child left the OR but died in the ICU. These were days for "ghosts."

SURVIVOR

NOT EVERYTHING WAS ENTIRELY LIFE and death, and so this is a discussion of *Survivor*, but a different kind.

When the TV show of *Survivor* came on, my family and I fell in love with every episode. We loved all the strategies and the alliances, and we talked about how we would play all of the puzzles. It was much fun. This was, and still is, a very fun show. Some years ago, I was talking with my wife about the game, and she said that if I sent in a video, I would be accepted for an interview. My understanding was that at that time, which was about the tenth season, the producers received several hundred thousand videos and only accepted a small number for interviews. My wife convinced me to go for it, which was a great struggle, given my very mellow personality, so we created a video lasting a few minutes.

I put on a scrub suit. I was already shaving my hair bald (didn't have much left anyway), and I had to describe three minutes about myself. You don't have much in three minutes, but I used a model of a brain, and then I begged the executive producer and creator of the show, Mark Burnett, to offer me a spot as I completed the audition with a pseudo-tattoo across my scalp that said, "SURVIVOR." It seemed über cool at the time, but we forgot about it after several months passed by and seemingly so did the *Survivor* train. Then one day after an early completion in the OR, I went with my wife and kids to the local mall. My wife was driving and suddenly her cell phone rang. A woman answered and asked for Mark. So there we were in the afternoon, and my wife's phone rang, the caller asking for me, using my first name. I looked at my wife, explaining I thought maybe it was from my patient, but I would have been called "Doctor" if that were the case.

I then took the phone and asked who was calling, and the caller said, "This is Penny Lane."

I said, "I'm sorry. I don't believe I know you."

And then she said, "It's Penny from *Survivor*."

I about lost control of my sphincters!

When Penny asked me who was with me, I told her my wife and children in our SUV. She then said to hang up and tell everyone that it was a mistake.

She then said, "We'll play a little phone tag, but we'll hook up," and she laughed a bit.

We got off the phone, and I started talking about this little "mistake" until the car stopped. I then grabbed my wife and told her that it was from *Survivor*.

The next morning at 5:00 a.m., California time, Penny called me, and we spoke on the phone for over an hour. She said that she and the producers really liked my video and, especially, my Brooklyn accent. She wanted to set me up for an interview. This meant that she was going to send me a long application that no one could see or read except my wife. It contained every job, all my income—including stocks, bonds, pensions, and bank accounts—every place I rented or owned, and basically everything about me, good or bad, that I knew existed. The way *Survivor* was done years ago was that if you lost the competition and were not on the jury, you went on a vacation but then returned to where they were producing the game and stayed there until it was over. This meant a lot of time because there were interviews with other TV stations after the game was completed, and this would be very difficult for me in a high-profile position.

I was also told that at the studio for my interview, I would sit in a room with my paperwork and not say a word to anyone, as they were all potential competitors.

I was sitting in this room, and several applicants were called, some staying longer than others had. I was entirely quiet, and then this young guy walked into our waiting area and looked at me and said, "Hey, Mark, what are you doing here?"

Everyone turned to look at me as if I was working as a covert operative for the Pentagon. It turned out that he was a friend and a former patient of mine. As he was a friend, he didn't say "Doctor," but he was wondering why I was at a television studio. He was a business owner who created commercials for his stores. I told him I drove with a friend to the studio and then tried to avoid any further discussion. It took a while before I could explain it to him.

Finally, I was called after a long wait. I told them that I had to tell three people at the clinic about the competition. They weren't very happy. They asked why I couldn't say some personal problem was going on, but I explained that would be difficult to reconcile after being on TV. I was told that most people lie, leave their jobs, or are already not working. They made me curse horribly because of my Brooklyn accent and wanted me to speak like that on the show. They discussed a lot of other issues, but telling my administrators at the clinic was a real red stop. This was good, because as we were getting closer, my wife and I were getting very nervous about doing it and the potential problems. It was a great deal of fun, getting excited for it, but I guess my day job was possibly too big a deal.

But maybe they would take a now-retired neurosurgeon?

SURVIVOR...A DIFFERENT KIND

OUT OF THE THOUSANDS OF patients I was privileged to care for over my career, many of the most exciting and breathtaking cases involved children. As I mentioned previously, I had a strong interest in the pediatric age group, and I almost pursued a subspecialty in pediatric neurosurgery. That being said, I worked at a clinic and hospital where we had a children's division associated with our general hospital. This offered an opportunity to care for a fair share of infants and children.

When I was a chief resident in Miami, I kept a diary of every case I consulted and operated upon as the primary surgeon. For Phase II of the Neurosurgery Board Certification, I had to prepare all of this information, including the diagnosis, radiology findings, and surgical procedures and results. This was presented prior to the final oral examination.

I didn't keep an ongoing diary throughout my career, but my memory remains honest and allows me to share some of these cases that will stay with me forever.

BACK FROM HOLIDAY

ONE WEEK I RETURNED FROM holiday and spoke to one of my associates about what had been happening in the department. I found out about an incredible case involving an infant with an AVM diagnosed while still in utero by using an ultrason. The ultrason is a device transmitting sonic waves that bounce against solid structures in the body. The baby's mother went into premature labor, and a caesarean section was performed emergently. The baby sustained a critical hemorrhage within the brain, causing a seizure and then a cardiac arrest. The baby was resuscitated but was quite ill. Before I returned to work, the baby had one more seizure and another cardiac arrest from which the baby recovered. My partner tried to transfer the baby to a pediatric neurosurgeon working at a university medical center, but the university was not speeding the process for the needed transfer. My partner discussed the case with our other associates, and no one, including me when I heard about it, was interested in pursuing surgery, which was more than likely going to result in death. I insisted on getting the patient to the university, but the pediatric neurosurgeon was reviewing all the images and records, and he was not ready to accept the transfer.

In my experience, when other professionals called me or my other partners regarding neurosurgical problems, we were always ready to help as soon as possible and immediately if the problem was an urgent one. This baby should have been transferred the first day my associate called the university.

Thursday of that week, I was operating on a serious head trauma case. I had continued my portion of the surgery involving reconstruction of the skull and repair of the dura and lacerated brain tissue. An oral-facial surgeon was completing a repair of many comminuted fractures of the facial bones. When this was completed, we would need to close the scalp opening, which was complex. While my associate in the OR was working and I was waiting to complete the final stages, an RN came into the OR, looking for me. One of my partners working in the OR across the corridor advised me that the baby was still in the neonatal ICU and had another cardiac arrest. Once again, the baby was recovered, and I was asked by my partner if I could do anything to help. My oral-facial surgeon told me not to worry, that he would complete the closure of the scalp without my assistance.

I then ran to the ICU and spoke with the parents and the pediatric intensivists. I had not met the family before, and I explained, as they already knew, that the baby was in very critical condition, and we had no further options but emergency surgery. I then had the baby transferred to the OR.

The baby was in a coma and was debilitated. I looked at the head, which was the size of a small melon. I needed to rearrange my thinking of the geometry of the brain, and I reviewed all the radiology imaging while the baby was being positioned for the surgery. I spoke with the surgical nurse, and we arranged for all of the instruments needed.

I have treated a fair number of AVMs over the years, but I had never attempted an AVM resection on an infant. For me, this was adjusting to the small dimensions of the brain and blood vessels. We started the case and opened the scalp and very thin skull over the area of the brain that we were going to incise. The brain was swollen, and I brought in the operating microscope. We used microsurgery, ultrason, stereotaxis, special metallic clips, several RNs, my physician assistant, and anesthesia for such a complex procedure. We found the blood clots within the deeper corridors of the brain chambers and then carefully, using precise microsurgery, we aspirated the clots. With this completed, we began to identify the AVM blood vessels that were deep in the brain and quite small. I cauterized and then resected the abnormal arteries and nidus (a new word we learned before) and completed with the final removal of the abnormal draining veins.

This surgery was completed after a little over six hours of work, but it was following five hours at the prior trauma-surgery case. That day involved a little over fifteen hours of work. The swelling of the brain was immediately resolved, and the brain was pulsing again, which is a very good sign. The vital signs were stable, and it appeared that we would get the baby out of the OR. One of the great concerns at this time was rebleeding by a remnant of the AVM or a significant stroke.

The baby remained stable following that night; we performed an X-ray of the arteries in the brain, and it appeared that the

AVM was completely resected and the blood clots were aspirated. There was no additional bleeding, and the infant appeared stable. The baby slowly improved, and ultimately the child was transferred from the ICU to the regular ward. The patient developed some increasing water within the brain, which we call hydrocephalus. This required the placement of a procedure called a ventriculoperitoneal shunting (VPS), which was performed by placing a specialized catheter into the enlarged cavities of the brain called the ventricles. The catheter then got attached to a magnetic-controlled pressurized valve that determined how much fluid was transferred to the abdomen (peritoneal). If you work as a pediatric neurosurgeon, it is common to perform eight (VPS) during a normal busy day, but then you have to add a ninth for repairing the malfunction of one of the earlier procedures performed during the day—a relatively simple procedure, but notorious for malfunctions and misadventures. It is all about plumbing. The baby was then sent home. The baby continued to get well, and several months later, one of our neurologists told me that the baby's examination appeared actually normal.

YOU AIN'T BEEN ON MY MIND

SEVERAL DAYS AFTER THE SURGERY, the professor of pediatric neurosurgery at the university telephoned my partner, who was originally taking care of the baby, to tell him that the university was ready for the transfer. My partner was very proud to say that I had operated on the child, and his X-rays were now much improved, with the baby now stable and getting better. The professor was very impressed that the infant had done so well, and he said he was surprised that such a complicated procedure could be performed outside of the university.

This is what I call "Pride and the Prejudice." As specialists of any kind, we all go to school for a long time and then to the university for resident training. I agree that if you are a professor at a university, you will see more cases than at most, but not all, clinics. In this particular case, if he was so concerned about who would care for the baby, why wasn't the baby transferred on day number one? It so happened that one specialist in our department was able to care for this baby without any assistance from the university. I would have been happier without the comment regarding the university, but that's my "Brooklyn" jumping out again. Despite my "Brooklyn," I found some "wings on angels."

HOW DID WE GET TO MAUI?

FOR OVER TWENTY YEARS, OUR family has vacationed to Maui in the Hawaiian Islands. It started when my wife and I left for Hawaii for a cruise ship holiday. Firstly, my wife is very seasick. Maybe, I should repeat—*very* sea sick. She was also in her fifth week of pregnancy, which translated to "first term," which is translated in most global dictionaries as "nausea and vomiting." We thought this was a great idea. She was desperately ill thinking about the trip to the airport. By the time we got to the cruise, I was certain I would need to ask the captain to call for a helicopter to get us toward the mainland. I begged, but it didn't work. The only thing that worked was when she got to Maui and was able to eat mashed potatoes and gravy from a Kentucky Fried Chicken franchise (my wife is southern). We eventually got home, but when we started thinking about our next holiday, we decided Maui was the way to go.

Hawaii has been our only trip, and we mix our casserole of Zen, a little pinch of Buddhism, an elephant tusk turned upward, and a main dressing of Judaism, Christianity, Islam, and any other dynamism to create peace and love. My hobby is physics and cosmology, but my thinking is particularly flexible.

For one holiday flight traveling to Los Angeles, it was delayed to Honolulu because of terrible weather. Our luggage made it ahead to Maui, but we lost our flight, and since this was the time of the typhoon near Japan, we had to wait three days to get to Maui! Everyone in our family was crying and miserable, believing much of our holiday was lost. I suddenly had a clue, and I phoned the concierge at our hotel on Maui. In fifteen minutes, we were in a taxi heading to a private airport. We found a plane with a pilot, copilot, and six additional seats. If we had any luggage, the plane would have traveled twice more, canceling Maui for the next two years. My youngest daughter noticed some masking tape throughout the plane, which got my attention, but I didn't mention it to anyone else. The pilots said that when the plane passed over the mountains in Honolulu, we'd encounter nasty weather again. The truth was that the day was perfect, and the climate was phenomenally calm and beautiful. We landed at a private airport where a white limousine was waiting for us. We packed the luggage from Honolulu that was now waiting on Maui and took off. We lost one day and had a perfect holiday. "Wings on angels!" I thought it was worth it!

LOST IN TRANSLATION

EVERY NOW AND THEN, WE ran into cases with unexpected diagnoses. This seemed to be one of my specialties. A patient came to see me at my office with a diagnosis of a tumor in the lower part of the spine. He had developed a problem with walking and control of his bladder function. He also had some numbness in his pelvis and legs.

When I examined him and reviewed his X-rays, it became clear that this large mass was compressing very important nerves attached to the spinal cord. He could develop partial or even thorough paralysis and lose sensation in his legs. His bladder and sexual function could be completely lost of all activity. The radiologists reviewing the MRI (magnetic resonance imaging) were convinced that the tumor was benign but in a difficult location. He would require extensive surgery in and around the spine.

On his day of surgery, we incised the lumbar spine region overlying the tumor and detached the muscles attached to the spine. We then opened part of the spine so that we could see the entire tumor mass. Looking at the tumor using microsurgery, I didn't recognize the type of tumor it was by the color and texture. Normally, we were expecting this tumor to belong to the meningioma class, schwannoma group, or ependymoma. The tumor was removed leaving a small remnant, because the size was intimately attached to the circuitry responsible for sphincter activity. The pathologist determined that this was a benign tumor, as expected, mostly found in the lungs and occasionally the brain, but never in the lumbar spine. Treating with steroids will often help to cure the diagnosis. The tumor was called sarcoidosis, and this allowed me to publish my last medical journal.

I did not sleep well before surgery. This has always been the case, and if it is a very difficult case, then I would be a true insomniac. It was impossible to determine how many patients or families asked me in the morning before a case started if I'd had a good night's sleep. I usually said that I'd had a few beer chasers before breakfast, so everything should go well. If I don't feel that humor is appropriate, I just say that I slept "like a baby." I have had to operate on many emergencies, when I seem to be at my best, because I just follow the blueprints in my own head, instead of staying up most of the night, thinking about the remedies. As I've said before, surgeons are sleep deprived.

When I was in training, we worked over one hundred hours/ week, at least in neurosurgery. Some years ago, the number of hours that a resident could cover changed dramatically. There were very dramatic rules and significant consequences if they weren't followed. Interestingly, for someone like me working in private practice at a clinic, each specialist of the four we had in neurosurgery was on call one week/month, following sequentially, one day at a time. We started on Friday morning, working until the following Friday morning. Occasionally, we changed the work schedule and sometimes, for example, I worked ten days straight, involving two weekends, at a trauma center where I worked in Wisconsin. No one controlled these arrangements but the neurosurgeons working. This was not controlled by anyone else, and neurosurgery made its own rules. I've had weeks where I was at home six hours over two days. The original argument for changing the call schedules for residents across the United States was to avoid errors from sleep deprivation. No one, however, really cared about my partners or me. The on call became far more adventurous with each new birthday! My last birthday cake was shaped as a call beeper.

SUNSHINE CAME SOFTLY THROUGH MY WINDOW

ONE EVENING WHILE ON CALL, I was sleeping, which in itself was a minor miracle, and the phone rang slowly after 1:00 a.m. My physician assistant called me and explained that an emergency was on its way and our sleeping, for the rest of the night, was now over.

It was a strange story indeed. A middle-aged man, who had been trained as an engineer and had been a functioning pilot, had a history of migraines that were treatable and never debilitating. He lived alone, and on the day before his calamity, he awoke in the morning with his right eye appearing fuzzy. He called his brother, who lived in another state, and he wondered if it was a migraine. The patient told him he didn't have any headaches, and he wasn't used to having any visual problems. The patient's brother told him to get to the hospital if it didn't improve.

The patient sat down in his family room and fell asleep. Over a period of several hours, he became completely blind in both eyes. He was blind and needed to get some help immediately. He managed to call a friend using his smartphone. His friend then drove him to our hospital where they sat together in the waiting area. Apparently, the receptionist did not understand that he became completely blind over twenty-four hours and misunderstood that he was already blind for several days. By the time he got into the ER, which was further hours later, the ER physicians understood, rather urgently, that this was a catastrophe.

My physician assistant called me about this adventure, and I ordered an immediate MRI. The MRI revealed a giant tumor of the pituitary gland called a mega-adenoma. This was not producing or deleting any hormones, but there was a hemorrhage that occurred within the tumor and caused it to enlarge, compressing both optic nerves (the nerves attached to the eyes and brain) and causing the recent blindness. The patient required emergency surgery, as the tumor was so large and the patient was now blind. I decided to open his skull to find the tumor and get the pressure off the optic nerves and the structures attached to the brain.

The patient was prepared for the surgery, but our conversation before the procedure was quite scary. I explained that his blindness appeared to be complete, without light coming into his vision, and that if any function returned, it would be quite impartial. He would probably require new arrangements for living. We even discussed braille, which I also mentioned to the patient's brother listening to us by phone. The patient and his brother wanted to know of these issues before he signed the consent.

The patient was given specialized medications and placed under general anesthesia. An incision was started in the scalp on the right side where the tumor appeared to be largest. The tumor was growing under both the right and left frontal lobes of the brain, for the tumor to compress both optic nerves. A wedge of bone was removed from the skull, and the dura was opened. At this point, we could see part of the front of the brain that was above the optic nerves and the important attachments to the undersurface of the brain, including some very critical blood vessels. This chamber of the brain region is a critical area, and removing the tumor involved a dissection and microsurgery that could easily lead to death with a slight misadventure. This was a great example of a benign tumor that gets quite a lot of attention, when we enter this neighborhood of the brain. We removed the entire tumor over a period of about five hours. The important critical structures remained intact, so it was now an issue of results.

With this book, I've tried to find the cases I will never forget. This is one of them, as this patient developed a return to normal functional vision within a month, improving almost on a daily basis. He returned to living at home after he left the hospital within two weeks. As I've said before, we found a lot of "wings" in that OR during several hours of that early morning.

HOLD ON TO WHAT YOU GOT

OVER THE YEARS, I'VE OPERATED upon many patients with trauma, and honestly, it's impossible to recall many of these individuals. However, several cases come to mind. Some injuries were quite horrific, and others were simply odd or bizarre.

The most critical and somewhat bizarre injury occurred when I was working as a chief resident in Miami and I was called to the ER. When I got to the critical trauma room for the worst types of injuries, I noticed a middle-aged woman lying on a bed with a lot of blood on her neck and chest. I asked the other physicians what had happened, and I was told that her husband had tried to decapitate her with a large carving knife, and the injury was almost completed. The patient was paralyzed from the shearing through the spinal cord, and the other trauma specialists had placed a tracheostomy cannula to support ventilation. The injury had almost gone from one side to the other and only some of the important blood vessels, on one side, remained intact and were normally circulating. The incredible aspect was that the patient would open and close her eyelids when questioned yes or no answers. I was stunned, and then I looked around the trauma room and asked what exactly they wanted me to do. I hadn't been trained to reattach a head, but the trauma specialists didn't know what else to do, so they figured that neurosurgery was a good place to start.

The brain was not obviously injured, and my first choice was to prevent the head from completely decapitating, so I placed some metallic tongs to the skull to create some traction, and this prevented any further movement of the head. I then called for a vascular specialist, and we brought the patient to the OR. Our goal was to try to reattach the critical blood vessels that were shorn apart, and this lasted for about thirty minutes before the patient had a cardiac arrest that couldn't be recovered.

The entire staff involved with this woman did everything possible to try and find some remedy. Had she lived, she would have been impaired in an almost unimaginable presentation, but we worked until we lost.

Some of us remember the talented actor and artist Christopher Reeve. He had sustained a tragic injury, not unlike this patient in the ER. Presuming the brain was still functioning, she would have lost all motor and sensory function below the head. Few understand that there are injuries affecting high levels of the spinal cord just below the brain that require the constant need for a respirator. The only available sensation would be determined by the pressure of the head, and the sensation of the muscles and face as well as some slight sensation from the scalp. There are surprisingly many patients with this degree of affliction. Many patients would beg for death, but amazingly, many find a way to see the light that is in their life. Christopher Reeve became a writer, producer, and director.

A ten-year-old was playing in his closet with the door closed. On the back of the door was a target for a dart game. The patient's brother and his friend were playing in the room, not knowing his younger brother was within the closet. The older brother then decided to throw a dart toward the target, exactly when the younger brother opened the door to come out. At that moment, the dart struck the ten-year-old in the middle of his forehead and deeply penetrated through the skull and into the brain. That resulted in surgery and a photograph for one of my trauma lectures.

I have encountered a pencil stuck in the brain after a fight between a couple of teenagers. I removed a large arrow from someone's head, a man who had been hunting in the woods, according to the sheriff's department, and one day a young man was working at a construction site when he leaned backward and struck an active pneumatic staple that discharged into the back of the brain. Injuries from fighting at bars were fairly common, with a well-earned mix of alcohol, guys and gals and pool tables, with pool cues. If I was called because of a fight with a pool cue, it meant, guaranteed, a crushed skull and a visit to my favorite cinema, also known as the OR.

THE DAYS OF WINE AND ROSES

SEVERAL YEARS AGO, A YOUNG man was driving his car, with his wife as a passenger in the shotgun seat and two children behind them, seated securely in the vehicle. Suddenly, the driver of the vehicle had a generalized seizure, which is a harrowing thing to see, and he became unconscious while still behind the steering wheel. The driver's wife leaned over and tried to gain control of the vehicle, which then crashed into another vehicle on the opposite side of the road. The driver of that vehicle, an elderly woman from a very successful family, died almost immediately. The driver recovered, and his wife was injured, involving many orthopedic insults. In the back seats, the twins were appropriately secured.

They were all transferred to the hospital, and the driver's brain CT revealed a tumor on the left side of the brain in the front of the temporal lobe. The position of the tumor was odd in shape and signal, and most specialists felt that it might be malignant, but we weren't certain. Other than the seizure, his examination was normal. He had had some emotional difficulties and anxiety during his wife's recent pregnancy. I was asked to see the patient, and ultimately I brought him to surgery. I found a benign tumor called a meningioma located in an odd position, and I was able to remove it completely, as best I could determine. He had no problems from the surgery, but unfortunately, his wife's injuries were taking a lot of time to heal. The children were not injured.

I subsequently became involved in a very bizarre legal issue when an attorney for the patient's wife sued the attorney of her husband. Regarding the patient who died, I made it clear that the seizure was entirely unexpected and could not be avoided despite just about any given circumstance. The attorneys were suing each other because one suggested that the driver's emotional disturbance and anxiety from the pregnancy could have led to a type of seizure that was not diagnosed by his psychiatrist, and this led to the seizure injuring my patient's wife. The wife was suing her husband's incompetent medical care, as per the psychiatrist, and anticipated money that would ultimately go to the husband and wife. This would also have a consequence regarding the woman, who passed during the trauma.

I explained seizures in the best way I could, and even though I was intimately involved with my patient and his family, I couldn't support this premise. My patient's attorney was hostile, and I was ready to translate some phrases from English to French to advise him of what I felt about everyone. As is usually the case, there was some settlement that was accepted by all involved. Good doctors, bad doctors. Good lawyers, bad lawyers.

WHO IS THE PRETTIEST
IN ALL THE LAND?

WHEN I ARRIVED AT WISCONSIN and was getting settled down, I was on call when a child fell from his bunk bed and crashed into a window in the bedroom. This was an eight-year-old, and because of the injury, a large shard of glass penetrated through the lower lumbar spine and into the sacrum. The trauma surgeon was originally called, as the glass could have torn into the rectum inside of the abdomen. Surgery would have involved placement of a rectum scope to make sure there were no injuries requiring repair. I was called in to see the patient for the spinal injury, but as I hadn't been in Wisconsin long, this trauma surgeon was a little "nervous." He then called the chief trauma surgeon, who told him that he'd already worked with me and that I was a pretty good surgeon. The surgeon in the ER wanted to transfer the child to the university, as the injury appeared complicated. When I saw the child and the X-rays, I knew that this would be a difficult case, but I was comfortable in treating the child. Transferring the child to the university would have taken over three hours, and I didn't think that was a good idea. The trauma surgeon suggested about three times that we should maybe transfer the patient, which was getting me slightly "pissed," remembering I'm from Brooklyn. I decided that the two of us should go to speak with the child's father and ask his opinion. The trauma surgeon discussed with the patient's father his concerns, and then I discussed mine, including some bad possible outcomes, and I offered the option of transfer to the university. The father then asked me if I felt if I could treat his child, and I said I believed I could do this, but it would be difficult. The father said almost immediately to do the best I could do, because he would prefer to remain at our hospital.

We went to the OR, and the scoping was completed, showing no injuries to the rectum or colon, and so the child was placed over to me. Interestingly, the trauma surgeon stayed in my OR for the entire procedure. Everything was prepped and ready to go, and then he saw me bring in my operating microscope. He then watched my microsurgery over the video scan as I found the glass shard and removed it very carefully. No nerves were damaged and the dura (seen in brain and spine) was repaired. The surgery took about four hours. The child walked out of the hospital in one week, without any impairment, including infection, which was a big concern. Before the child left the hospital, the trauma surgeon came to find me and told me he would always give me the benefit of the doubt, and he apologized in questioning my skills.

This was great, that everything went well, but what if there had been some problem? A number of complications could have presented, and I suspect that the rewards would have been very different. You have to learn to work with people and have the appropriate faith. If a physician provides marginal care, it will become obvious, and it will be addressed appropriately. I was happy that I earned a friend, but I didn't make it entirely easy on him, as I decided to be a bit of a pain in his ass, but in a friendly way.

FADED PHOTOGRAPHS

I HAVE A LOT OF photographs of my patients and me. The vast majority involved great results, but there exist some losses. I've lost people for expected reasons, but some for unexpected reasons.

Years ago, I met an eighteen-year-old girl who became quite ill with a malignant tumor located in the back of the brain, called the cerebellum. This tumor is called a medulloblastoma, and it carries a poor prognosis. She developed too much pressure in her brain because of the tumor invading and compressing upon the brain. She had symptoms of headaches, vomiting, double vision, poor gait, and coordination. This is often found in children where the results are more problematic, but on occasion, we find this tumor in adults where they tend to do better. We planned to pursue surgery and then follow with chemotherapy and radiation.

We performed the surgery, and my impression was that any part of the brain that appeared malignant was surgically removed. This meant that, looking at the affected brain under the operating microscope, I could see that the residual brain was grossly normal looking, but it didn't mean that invasive tentacles weren't around. She healed beautifully and had her chemotherapy, which she supported without issues. She then had her radiation. This type of cancer easily spread throughout other areas of the brain and even into the spine. The pathologists believed that if we could get past five years without any recurrence, we might be able to talk of cure. This sweet girl went off to college, and her follow-ups were great with her neuro-oncologist and me. The radiation oncologist was also very happy. At five years, she had a normal-looking MRI, and she appeared to have a normal neurologic examination. I was thrilled, and I started looking for my "wings."

Six months later, I was called to see her lying on a bed in the neurosurgery ward. She was again as sick as she had been when I first met her five-and-a-half years ago. She'd had a new MRI, and this had demonstrated a recurrent large tumor in the same area of her original surgery. I was devastated. I took her to surgery again, in the same area, but this time we found something different. Radiation is a plus and a minus. It can heal, and it can hurt. Radiation can alter the DNA (deoxyribonucleic acid) and cause the appearance of a new tumor that is almost always malignant and generally very nasty. At the OR, I pursued a radical resection of a new cancer called a glioblastoma. This is the most nefarious of any brain malignancy and always without a cure. She didn't want any further treatments of chemotherapy. She would come by to visit with me, and I believe she was there to teach me. She taught me a little more about life than I knew or understood. She became strong as her illness followed the "ghosts." We lost her in another year.

Somewhere is a photograph of a pretty young lady holding my shoulders with both of us smiling.

JASON AND THE ARGONAUTS

I REMEMBER MY FIRST NEUROSURGICAL case, which was the removal of what we term a subdural hematoma. This is often heard on TV and in movies. One hears of life-and-death situations, but until you are in that reality, it is entirely impossible to understand what that really means. I can say that if you do this long enough, eventually you find yourself working in the most complicated life-and-death situations imaginable, but your work is a total focus on the task at hand. Earlier during my career, I would be working on a very difficult surgical crisis that would clearly be recognized as a life-and-death phenomenon, and I would struggle between recognizing that one small mistake could cause death or devastation. No one ever sat me down to discuss any of these considerations. You were generally expected to find your pass to the mountaintop by reading through the legends on Mount Olympus.

During my training, most neurosurgeons found they were better skilled at taking care of children or engaging in the extreme adventure of aneurysm and AVM surgery. Some were very proficient at trauma surgery or spine surgery. Some surgeons enjoyed taking out tumors. Somewhere, you need to determine not what you do well, but what you don't do well. If you have the ego, then you need to make sure that the patient is in a safe place, if it isn't with you. That is a hard lesson, and some never learn the right answers.

THE GOLDEN FLEECE

NOT LONG AGO FROM THIS writing, a young woman in her thirties was referred to me. She had undergone two small leakages from a small aneurysm blister. Her first bleeding was a history of a horrible sudden headache, but as she had a history as a chronic pain patient, she was given medication and sent home from the ER she original visited. The next episode was a returning sudden and severe headache that led to a CT scan of the brain, revealing that she had sustained a small, what-we-call "sentinel leakage." This leads to a very miniscule leakage of blood around the aneurysm blister but closes off before a monstrous hemorrhage can occur. Blisters on an aneurysm are very dangerous because of the small size, making it difficult to clip by surgery. Using the coiling technology, called endovascular surgery, was considered a problem as well, because of the small size of the blister. We thus planned to clip the aneurysm by open surgery and exploring the aneurysm directly. Just before the procedure, I reviewed the case with a resident in general surgery, who was going to assist me, with my physician assistant. I explained that the greatest concern was the size of the blister and that this could lead to a calamity.

In the OR, the general anesthesia was started, all of the appropriate medications were given, and the patient was positioned for the incision. The incision was made on the left side, the side of the aneurysm and also the side of the speech circuitry. The bone wedge was removed and the left frontal lobe was identified. My next step was slowly compressing the frontal lobe, using specialized brain retractors to identify the deeper structures of the brain in order to identify the aneurysm. As I started to retract the frontal lobe, we encountered an inundation of bleeding, and we were in serious trouble.

When working on aneurysms, you must identify the part of the aneurysm that is attached to the artery containing the blister and then the segment of the artery immediately beyond the aneurysm. This allows for a very important proximal (before) and distal (after) control. While we were trying to move the left frontal lobe, the blister was stuck to the undersurface of the brain, and it burst open before we could identify any of this anatomy, proximal or distal. I got the brain retractor in position, but the bleeding continued, and the blood pressure was dropping precipitously. I brought the operating microscope in position and then tried to stop the bleeding so that I could find the aneurysm, which was hemorrhaging. At one point, the blood pressure was so low that a cardiac arrest was called, even though it wasn't a full arrest since there was still bleeding in the brain. If the brain is bleeding, the heart is pumping.

All the drapes were removed and three anesthesiologists were trying to strengthen the pulsations and try CPR. During all this work, I stood as quietly as possible beside my microscope and finally identified the aneurysm. I was able to position a clip on the aneurysm, but I certainly didn't feel secure about the situation. Once the clip was situated, all the bleeding stopped completely, and the blood pressure started to recover nicely. Infection was an issue, because of all of the doctors in the OR at the same time. Despite the catastrophe, I did my work and didn't talk to anyone while all the chickens lost their heads and were running around the OR. I performed my surgery and saw only one thing—getting the bleeding stopped and finding the aneurysm to get it clipped safely. Ultimately, the blood pressure was allowed to elevate, to make sure that the aneurysm was secure, without any further bleeding. The patient completely stabilized, and we all looked at each other thinking, Holy shit! That was clearly from Brooklyn.

The aneurysm was remedied, the circulation throughout the brain was safe, and the patient left the hospital in less than two weeks. The day she left the hospital, she saw me walking around the ward, and she ran over to me, hugged me, and told me, while crying, "Thanks for saving my life."

No question about it—this earned some "wings on a few angels." I still have a lot of trouble dealing with the notions of life and death. It was a good day, and she went on with the rest of her life, her not forgetting me and me not forgetting her.

WHAT DO YOU GET WHEN YOU FALL IN LOVE?

MY FIRST OPPORTUNITY AS AN assistant in neurosurgery was in Liege, Belgium when I watched, in awe, as my professor successfully treated a ruptured aneurysm in the brain. This was performed with microsurgery, which I had never seen previously, and as I've stated before, the ambiance in the OR was beyond compare. I didn't understand most anything I was watching, but I did recognize it was special. When the procedure was completed, the professor, who was fifty-eight years old at the time, stated in French, "Les anevrysmes sont toujours l'aventure," which translates into "aneurysms are always an adventure."

I never had a mystery, regarding the internal compass chasing after me. I was meant to become a physician, and I was fairly certain that it would somehow involve the nervous system. That one day in the OR was a final seduction, but listening to a chief of neurosurgery remain in a continued dreamlike sense of amazement, as if he were within a magical crystal ball, was in itself breathtaking. My understanding of this, at the age of twenty-five, was very foggy. Connections are often made in strange ways and stay with you for no obvious reasons. In this particular situation, I recall turning sixty years old, which allowed for a little celebration. I thought of many things in my life, but one that weighed heavily was my professor's statement. Those few words meant everything to me as a neurosurgeon. I fully understood that the work never really ends and you can never take anything in the slightest for granted.

How do you describe an unforgettable poem, play, or book? What of the music of a melody, or a lyric, that tumbles tears from your eyes? What of work well done, regardless of the type? What is belief? What is faith? What is love?

AROUND THE WORLD IN EIGHTY DAYS

SOME TWENTY YEARS AGO, I was asked to consult with an eighty-eight-year-old physician. He had sustained a massive hemorrhage within the brain and was in a coma. The patient's family wanted to discuss all of the medical issues and options. I demonstrated the CT scans of the brain, and I explained that, given the size of the hemorrhage, his clinical examination, and his age, I found it very difficult to advise a major brain surgery.

I then found myself waiting over two hours for a decision. I was already aggressive regarding my "hawkish" attitude for surgery, but I still had lessons to learn. The family decided to transfer the patient to the hospice ward, which is a nonaggressive approach for medical care. Whatever the reasons—envy, greed, faith, belief, love, or God—these are all real reasons, and most importantly, there are no right or wrong answers. Why is surgery at eighty better than eighty-eight if the conditions were fairly much the same?

JULES VERNE I

ONE WEEKEND I BROUGHT MY wife and children to celebrate at a wedding reception. It was a lot of fun, and my wife and I always enjoyed dancing together. I knew many of the invitees, and so I was busy in conversation, generally talking about my work. People always liked talking about my work because there seems to exist a sort of science fiction nature to it. As usual, when sixty-year-olds started knocking on the door to ask about my eventual retirement, I found it odd, that this wasn't really about my personal retirement. Unless my life starts to resemble a dimensionless emptiness, I will hope that my life finds a collection of children growing, living, and maturing. There will be love, tears, and everything in between. They'll be grandchildren scrapping the sidewalks.

When my dad was healthy and we had him for a while, he had a talk with me that I hadn't thoroughly understood. He had some success but retired too soon and rejected the whole process of retirement. He told me that after retirement, what really is there holding your time? For him, his friends constantly thought about getting ill and dying.

I've never wanted to stop working because work is living.

There is work, and there is holiday. When you retire, despite the reason for the retirement, you can't look at some void. It may certainly not seem obvious at first, but you have to look with great spirit. Look for love, peace, friendship, and hope. Look for prayer, whoever or however you define that to be. Life is doors, curtains, and seeking beneath that which is hidden from us. Life is and has always been a "Mysterious Island."

WHITE JACKET, WHITE JACKET

THERE IS A WHITE JACKET that is a good one and a bad one. A bad one is when the patient sees a "Dr." on the white jacket and gets nervous, agitated, sweaty, and elevated blood pressure. A good response is when the doctor wears the white jacket and is under the impression that somehow there exists an inherent safety zone, because it says "Dr." on the jacket. While I was being checked over by an RN for an insurance contract, my blood pressure was fairly high, 194/110. This was repeated several times, and the recordings continued elevated. I was athletic, thin, and a nonsmoker.

Somewhere those little things called genes and chromosomes were sneaking up on me. I made an appointment with one of my internists. Now working like Sherlock Holmes, he also identified that he would find most everything abnormal, including a high lipid profile and diabetes, requiring oral medications. The older you get, the more pills you wind up taking in the morning and evening. My internist advised that after some years, I'd be on insulin because of my pancreas slowing down. This is what we call type 2 diabetes. Eventually, my blood sugars got worse, and I started insulin. I've had many patients over the years with diabetes and treating with insulin. I always told my patients that the insulin is better and easier to use. I, of course, was lying like a dog and hated every bit of it. Diabetes is a rather serious affair, and you have to watch the blood sugars and take the medications like "Brooklyn." After all, I was wearing a white jacket!

SUNRISE, SUNSET

I CONTINUED TO WORK HARD and often took more emergency on call than my partners. If they needed extra days or evenings off, I was often ready to take the extra work. I was not seeking a bonus, but so much of my work starting from Miami and beyond kept me busy with being on call that I didn't mind working. One evening, my wife and I were talking about my additional work, and I agreed we needed to find a better solution. At that point, my phone rang, and my mom got on the phone to tell me that my dad had had a cardiac arrest. He was resuscitated and transferred to his hospital in Florida. We travelled down to Florida and found my dad unresponsive because of his extended loss of oxygen. The cardiac muscle function was quite weak, and it appeared to be a difficult situation for the family and me. Everyone agreed that my father would not tolerate a partial improvement and find himself living in an impaired and debilitated situation. I then wore two hats, one as a doctor and one as a son. I wasn't prepared for any of it. Ultimately, we sent my dad to hospice where he left this life while my hands held his own and my sisters touched him for his final voyage. The last thing he said to me was only two days before he became ill. We talked for a while, and then he said, "I love you." Wings? Ghosts?

QUE SERA, SERA

ONE AFTERNOON, I WAS LECTURING a group of physical medicine and rehabilitation specialists as well as therapists. I truly enjoyed lecturing and had a lot of photographs to present to my audience. I presented lectures to other recipients on aneurysms and many bizarre trauma cases. For this particular case, I had photographs of every segment of this procedure. A photographer was in the OR and demonstrated how the patient was positioned and where I stood to place the sterile drapes at the beginning of surgery. I demonstrated making the initial incision and the stages of each segment of the dissection. We identified the spine and then brought in the operating microscope, which was nicely viewed with the magnification. I showed the removal of the bone spurs from the vertebrae and removal some very degenerated discs from the spine. I then showed the reconstructed spine using hardware and cadaver bone as well as other substitutes. The surgery had been completed after three hours. When I completed the surgery, I announced to the audience that, given the number of hours, over the many years of this surgery, I was probably going to develop very degenerative disease of my own spine. It turned out that within a couple of years, I had the same surgery performed on me, without the photographs. Following that surgery, I was unable to turn my neck to the right for an entire year. The joints in part of my spine were "over distracted," and it took quite a bit of my own therapy to get well again.

JULES VERNE II

BACK TO THE WEDDING (REMEMBER when I went to the wedding with my wife?), the following Monday, I was in the OR reconstructing a very degenerated cervical spine. The patient was very large and weighed up to three hundred pounds. I had to lean over the operating table, which was difficult for me. I also had my own spine problems with reconstruction in my cervical spine and degenerative-lumbar spine disease. Surgeons often learn that as they get older, they get smarter and can control their surgical skills more masterfully. The problem is that we generally don't physically advance like our cerebrums (brains). We get smarter, but we can't stand at the operating table!

I completed my work and then went to the surgeon's lounge to dictate the procedure I had just performed. I got dressed into my usual clothes and went to my office. Two weeks before, I had cared for my last aneurysm patient. This gentleman in his seventies was visiting with his family, as he did most every summer. He and his family normally live in St. Louis. While he was boating, he had an aneurysm burst in his brain on the left side. He had some language difficulties, but they were very temporary and reversible. The bleeding had stopped, and he was stable, but based on the location and shape of the aneurysm, it was recommended to operate by open surgery and place a clip on the aneurysm. He had one aneurysm that bled, but every now and then, a patient will have more than one aneurysm, as was the case with this patient. The other aneurysms could be treated by the endovascular treatment and had not yet bled, thus the risk for bleeding in the aneurysms not yet treated was certainly lower than the aneurysm that did bleed, requiring surgery. As he and the rest of his family lived in St. Louis, we decided to transfer him back home. He did beautifully from his surgery in Wisconsin, and we agreed he was well enough to return home by vehicle. My surgery on the patient weighing three hundred pounds reminded me of "Journey to the Center of the Earth." After my surgery on that cervical spine patient, I was planning to talk with the neurosurgeon planning to transfer my patient to St. Louis for the definitive treatments.

GHOST AT THE GAS STATION

WHEN I GOT BACK TO my office, the other surgeon, from St Louis, wasn't available and when I looked at my computer scan, it appeared a bit unclear but not horribly so. I had a headache after my surgery from the morning case, and so I complained, to myself, that I was tired. When you are a surgeon, you always have reasons to be fatigued. I decided to head on home. I then went to a gas station where I had visited thousands of times and positioned my car in front of a fuel pump. I got out of my car, looked at the fuel pump, and was certain that I had just landed at NASA. I did not know how to use my credit card, or if I needed to pay with cash. I was confused, but interestingly, I didn't recognize that I was in trouble.

There was a very nice young man, working at the service market next to the fuel pumps. He approached me and asked me if I needed some help. I explained that I was having difficulty with my credit card, and he said that occasionally that happens, and he corrected using the card for me. I then tried to give him money, but he told me it was already completed. The "ghosts" were weighing a bit heavier, but as usual, I was in complete denial.

Whenever I return home from the hospital or clinic, no matter what the time is, I call my wife. This time, I did not call her when I returned home. I got home before she did, and the children stated I was tired and wanted to rest for a while. Later that evening, when I got up from my snooze, we had a talk, and my wife felt something was wrong. Everything about my conversation was perfect, but I started to talk about a sofa in our bedroom and kept using the wrong word. She asked me a lot of questions, and all of them were correct. She placed me in bed and figured she would watch me very closely. The following day, I had surgery scheduled, but my wife convinced me to take the day off and rest. This was something I never did.

LOST IN THE CLOUDS

I TRIED TO PHONE THE hospital. I realized almost immediately that I didn't have the slightest idea what the phone number was, and it seemed as if I was floating within a "ghost." I looked at my wife and started to cry. I realized I was in serious trouble. My wife called one of my neurologists, also a friend, and he told her to get us to the hospital closest to our home. This was not the same trauma facility where I worked, but I knew most of the physicians and many of the nurses and technologists working at this fairly new hospital.

I was brought to the ER and found myself lying on a table looking up, at a large contingency of people. I was now wearing one of those new Dior pajamas, of course, a pure fantasy, probably reflecting the consequence of the stroke.

My blood sugar was very high, as was my hemoglobin A1C, another important parameter for diabetes. The week before we went to the wedding, I was struggling with an infected root canal and as antibiotics were not resolving the inflammation and pain, my dentist extracted the tooth. The tooth was at the back of the mandible and would not have a cosmetic or functional impairment. An infection in the oral cavity is, however, a potential source of disease spreading to the blood or up to the cranium. I've learned that many oral surgeons are far more conservative, regarding surgical interventions for root canal disease. My blood pressure was around 100 systolic. Normally, for someone my age, with hypertension, internists suggest keeping the systolic (upper) number on the blood pressure scale to the lower side. This helps to avoid arteriosclerosis, or thickening, of the arteries. For people with strokes in their medical history, we like the systolic numbers to stay higher, between somewhere in the 120s to the lower 150s during the acute phase of the stroke. The blood pressure can then be lowered as the stroke is stabilized. I was thus in a poor triangle of oral infection, low blood pressure, and a rather disturbed diabetes that was the poor consequence of my (bad) white jacket.

I was sent to the CT scan of the brain that revealed episodes of what we call a watershed infarct. I had two on the left, which was the recent event, and an older one on the right-hand side.

Ischemia involves a decrease of circulation without hemorrhage. Depending upon the location and density of the known structures, the identification of the functional loss may be determined. A reversal of the impairment, lasting one to two hours, would be termed a transient or reversible loss. Infarction is an irreversible loss of function. My impairment was called watershed because of the location of the circulation loss and was an irreversible ischemia or infarction. This was determined by the images on the scans and my loss of function.

When I looked at my CT scan, despite my acute impairment when I was hospitalized, I was able to identify the anatomy and pathology seen on the scans as I had always done. I looked at my wife, and my second set of tears told me "no wings" for that day. I realized that I would never work as a neurosurgeon again. My greatest fears had also been the health of my family and the loss of my work—no hobbies such as chess, golf, or other fun things to keep us busy. I liked reading and watching sports on TV, but this is not a form of life for someone used to running at a velocity approaching light speed. I found myself hypnotized by an empty space, and it was far from comfortable.

I was transferred to a room, and I underwent the usual stroke work-up. I had a specialized MRI, electrocardiogram with stress echo, and treadmill stress test. I also had ultrason testing, as to be expected with a cardiac workup. The heart appeared healthy, but I needed to get the blood pressures higher. The biggest struggle was getting my diabetes healthy, which took many months. I take oral medications for diabetes twice a day and insulin twice a day. My friends, the neurologists who I've known for years, were now testing me as I've seen done thousands of times in the past.

SAILING AWAY

WHEN MY COGNITION SLOWED DOWN, I was trying to understand what was impaired and why. I understood all my colors, but there were many other problems. I clearly had some control with right and left and repeating some questions, such as take your right thumb and touch your left ear and then your right knee. That was extremely difficult and had to be done slowly for me to get it right, and it was still not a certainty I'd get it right. I would confuse a pencil and pen, and many vocabulary words appeared lost to me. This was my "ghost" and stayed with me for months. I started to work with a speech therapist shortly after I left the hospital.

STILL SAILING AWAY

THE THERAPIST EXPLAINED THAT MUCH recovery would occur after time had passed. I started studying many worksheets, including vocabulary, synonyms and antonyms, and word scrambling. I worked for many days, getting better over time. Some days I felt extremely frustrated, and I didn't believe that anything positive was happening. During my early therapy, I envisioned the anatomy of my injuries and pictured the structures of the brain. I've studied quite a lot of neuropathology and sectioned and studied the segments of the brain in the pathology department. I began seeing this again in my own mind. My goal was to help the injured area of stroke get healthier and facilitate the adjacent healthy brain to get it stronger. Time helped, puzzles helped, and in particular, memory was very important. At one point, I could repeat eight numbers in a row, front and back, and eight words, front and back. I found that some activities were easier than others were, but if the speed of some activities was too rapid, I would struggle. It was a bit like French when I was first learning. At the beginning, it was very difficult for me to watch a French movie, but I got more fluent over time. I'm going to include a few of my worksheets that kept me busy every day.

SCRAMBLED SENTENCES

- Joking you must be (sounds like Yoda the Jedi Master from Star Wars)
- Slept they noon until
- Me call six at
- You here shouldn't be
- Time up to get

These are only five sentences that are scrambled, but I reviewed hundreds until it came to me almost one day. I sat down and started working with a new worksheet, and suddenly it was clear and understandable. It remained as such, but I couldn't find some arrow to direct me.

YES/NO QUESTIONS

Do you hang a picture on the ceiling?
Do you sit on a sofa?
Do you put butter on ice cream?
Are locusts a type of bird?

Again, I've been through hundreds of these questions.

FILL IN THE LETTERS FOR THE STATES

N-BRA-K-; -R-ZON- -OW-; I-LI-O-S -EN-S-LVA-I-.

This is an example going through some of the states, but it exists for furniture, foreign nations, weather conditions, colors, transportation, clothing, and animals. I've had friends with advanced degrees make mistakes, with many of these being "forced errors." I've had some want to argue with my therapist. You know who you are.

As weeks were going by, I was improving rapidly, and at three months, my speech therapist believed that she couldn't assist me any further. This didn't mean I was where I wanted to be personally, but my therapist did not know how to improve my results. As a therapist, she had never worked with a neurosurgeon, and as my vocabulary picked up, she gave me medical journals to review and discuss, which seemed to help.

At the start of my therapy, I would sit at one end of the table, and my therapist would place a large rubber band, a pencil, a pen, a sheet of papers and a paper clip, on the table in front of both of us. My therapist would then give me restrictions such as place the paper clip over the sheets of paper, then move the rubber band to the left side of the pencil. We would then go through many potential options and at different speeds. The faster the instructions were, the more difficult the task to complete.

At the beginning of my therapy, I couldn't call a "button" correctly or, similarly, a "curtain" or a "bucket." I would be given a photograph with people and items on the street or inside a supermarket, and I would have to identify everything in the photograph including clothing, accessories, foods, colors, hardware, and items from outside the supermarket. Children, with young brains to develop and mature, have brain function known as plasticity. This allows the dense circuitry within the brain to vary in cerebral functioning. This suggests that some functions of the brain are being prepared for speech or motor function, but a severe injury can change the function, to a degree, while the brain is growing. This is most dramatic with infants and children, but we are learning about this with adults, after strokes and trauma. I struggled mightily with all of my therapy and work on the Internet, and my results went from 40% correct to close to 100%. After about six months, most people speaking with me had no idea I'd had a stroke. I make mistakes each and every day, but I've learned how to slow down my talking and change vocabulary words when I can't find the one I'm looking for.

When I talk, I sense that there is an occasional hesitancy when speaking, and often I seem to be the only one aware of the mental stuttering. I'm not sure that this will change dramatically from where my verbal skills are at this time. My memory was always excellent. My verbal difficulties did not take my surgery skills away from me, but it required some time to synchronize it all. I knew every instrument I needed on the OR table, but if

I hadn't reviewed everything, I would be able to pick out what I needed and make it work as always. Of course, the bar is very high when you're a neurosurgeon and I opted to retire, after almost twenty-nine years of private practice. Attorneys, experts working in medical liability, and many administrators decided that it was time to try and fill the space in our beautiful sky.

Sailing, sailing away…

EPILOGUE:
YOU CAN'T ALWAYS GET WHAT YOU WANT, BUT IF YOU TRY SOMETIME, YOU'LL GET WHAT YOU NEED

WITH WHATEVER IT IS THAT we choose for a career, it is extremely important that we don't ignore how young we are when the disability agents come looking for you. Most professionals, physicians or not, get very unthoughtful about controlling our well being. Professional athletes have great insurance carriers that are generally paid for by the athlete's agents. This is how it works from them. This would also be true for musicians, artists, and singers. For others, you are generally not worrying about your income when you are young. This is a huge mistake. For physicians, most worry about life insurance, term or not, but very important. It is a great idea to have a strong disability term. Be smart and be careful!

I've been so very fortunate to find my calling so early in my life and be ready to open any door, finding my way toward the top of my mountain. I've had many "angel wings" and a few "clouds" and "ghosts" around some hidden shadows. So many doors, can open, or *close*, during a lifetime. While studying in Miami, I was fully prepared to continue my work as a pediatric neurosurgeon, with many potential options, but I decided upon a different path, following an unknown distant highway.

I have treated thousands of patients and have loved so many, from infants through nonagenarians (aged in the nineties), but not, of course, forgetting our baby afflicted while still "in utero."

Many dreams grew forth from the wishes of a young boy carrying a doctor's kit, to reading such marvelous books about my heroes. Eventually, I carried a real "black bag" and wore a good white jacket. One day, someone told me I was now a doctor of medicine, and that will never change.

For not working, in academics at a university, I managed to get my name in several medical journals, and I found my name in a few varieties of Who's Who.

In central Florida, on my first day of work, I met a young, beautiful, twenty-two-year-old who also happened to be the smartest and most wise lady I've ever met. As much as I have had and as much as I have lost, I've had my girl who has always kept me looking forward to the sun. She is the love of my life, my best friend, and the mother of our six children.

To end my story, there is absolutely no way I can adequately thank my patients at my side. What a thrill and privilege. There is clearly no other comparison.

49200493R00078

Made in the USA
Lexington, KY
29 January 2016